PLANT BASED DIET COOKBOOK FOR BEGINNERS

365 DAYS OF BUDGET-FRIENDLY & EASY-BREEZY RECIPES FOR A TRULY HEALTHY APPROACH TO LIFE & FOOD. RESPECT YOUR HEALTH & CHANGE YOUR ROUTINE | 28-DAY MEAL PLAN

RACHEL VITALE

Table of Contents

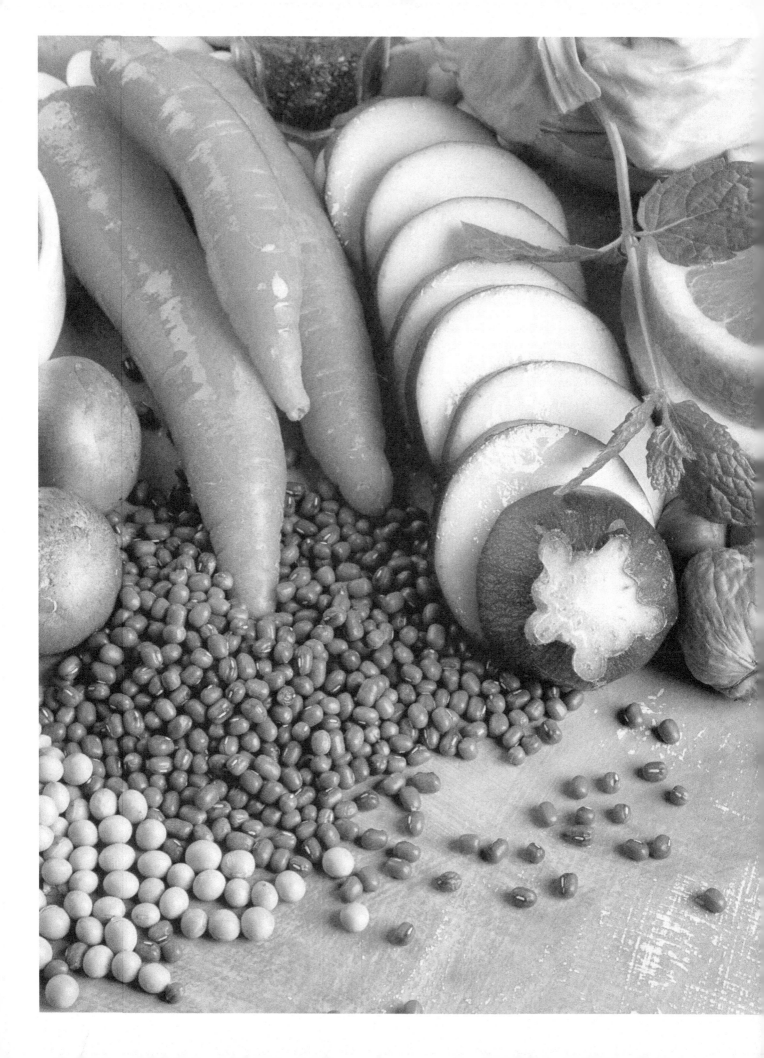

Introduction

There are many reasons for following a plant-based diet, from reducing meat in your diet overall to implementing one or two "meat-free days" each week. If your current diet is meat-heavy, this will take some major adjustments, so it is best not to make the switch from red meats to full veganism overnight. Veganism or vegetarianism works best when whole, natural foods are chosen instead of packaged or processed options. A lot of marketing is involved in promoting meat-free packaged snacks and condiments. However, many of these may contain sugars, high amounts of sodium, artificial color, additives, and other ingredients.

When making a leap from other diets to plant-based diets, anything can happen along the way. Of course, there are instances where you might fall off the wagon and turn to animal-based diets or processed foods. However, what you should understand is that it is normal to fall and regress occasionally. The transformation is not easy; therefore, forgive yourself for making mistakes here and there. Concentrate on the bigger picture of living a blissful life where you are at a lower risk of cancer, diabetes, and other ailments. More importantly, keep yourself inspired by connecting with like-minded people. Do not overlook their importance in the transition, as they face the challenge you are facing.

In conclusion, there is no surprise that a vast argument claims that the plant-based diet is either a vegan one (which is plant-focused) or vegetarian (which accommodates some animal foods). Both cases are incorrect. The plant-based diet uses plants, and it strongly rejects processed foods like white rice and added sugars. On the other hand, vegan and vegetarian diets allow some processed foods.

This book's primary goal is to present plant-based recipes in their most wholesome forms. The cookbook seeks to guide beginners on the plant-based diet. It will help you appreciate the essentials of whole-based plant foods through giving flexible options and various cooking combinations.

To be successful in dieting, all that needs to be done is to stick to the plan. It may seem extremely confusing and difficult at first, but any diet will become easier with practice. As long as the basic guidelines of a plant-based diet are followed, you will become healthier in no time! The secret is to start small; remember that you have no reason to make huge changes overnight. Even simply changing one meal this week to a plant-based recipe will already be a step in the right direction!

Chapter 1: What Is a Plant-Based Diet?

A plant-based diet is based on eating whole plant foods. This means you will be cutting out all highly refined foods like oil, refined sugar, and bleached flour. On top of cutting these foods out, you will also begin to minimize or exclude how much egg, dairy products, and meat you eat! Instead, you will be able to enjoy whole grains, vegetables, fruits, tubers, and all types of legumes

The most common reason why folks make this switch is to lose weight. Truthfully, there is a great deal of logic in doing so. Many individuals try their hardest to lose weight, yet they seem to come up short. And, while many factors go into losing weight, the fact of the matter is that, often, there is a need to make a radical switch in eating habits.

The first step to following a whole food plant-based diet is understanding what it means. To put it plainly, it means filling the majority of your diet with foods that are not processed or refined and come directly from plants. They are foods that are as close as possible to their source and are completely unmodified. It is not a diet restricted solely to fruits and vegetables; there are many delicious alternatives to help you have a satisfying choice of foods to eat.

In addition to eating fruits and vegetables, a whole food diet also includes eating various whole grains. Care should be taken when you choose your grains, however, as not all whole grains are as "whole" as they sound. When you choose the right grains, you can reap the benefits of complex carbs and vital vitamins and nutrients, adding taste, texture, and proper nutrition to your diet.

Grains are found in the seeds of various grasses. They can be found in wheat, oats, rice, cornmeal, and barley. Grains are considered "whole" when their three parts - bran, germ and endosperm - are intact. When they are processed, they are stripped of bran and germ and other vital nutrients. This results in refined and enriched grains, which make products such as white bread and white rice have a longer shelf life. These foods, as you probably know, are not so healthy for you. When you read product labels, look for the words refined or enriched grains and steer clear. In refined grains, the lost nutrients are never replaced. Though the products are fortified with the stripped nutrients, it does not provide the same benefits as eating whole foods with the natural nutrients right from the start.

Health Benefits of a Plant-Based Diet

Better Nutrition

Plants are healthy to eat, but most people fail to eat the appropriate number of veggies and fruits; therefore, following a plant-based diet will boost your productivity. Vegetables and fruits are filled with antioxidants, vitamins, fiber, and minerals. Based on studies, fiber is a nutrient that most people do not get nearly enough, even though it comes with tons of healthy perks—it is good for the heart, waistline, blood sugar, and the gut.

Weight-Loss

When following a plant-based diet, people tend to have a lower body mass index (BMI) than people on an omnivorous diet. However, research shows that you will be more successful at dropping pounds and keeping them off when you follow a plant-based diet.

Healthier Hearts

Following a plant-based diet is likely to reduce the risk of cardiovascular diseases and lessen other risk factors of heart disease by reducing cholesterol and blood pressure and enhancing blood sugar control. Following a plant-based diet can also help quell inflammation, which increases the risk of heart disease by regulating plaque buildup in the arteries.

Lower Diabetes Risk

Irrespective of your body mass index (BMI), following a plant-based diet, lowers the risk of diabetes. Another study, published in February 2019, states that you tend to have higher insulin sensitivity when you follow a plant-based diet, which is significant for maintaining a healthy blood sugar level.

Reduces the Risk of Cancer

The consistent consumption of adequate legumes, veggies, fruits, and grains is associated with a lower cancer risk. Disease-fighting phytochemicals found in plants are known to prevent and halt cancer. Studies also indicate an association between the consumption of processed meats and a rise in cancer risk, especially colorectal cancer.[1] Therefore, there are benefits from consuming more plants and choosing healthy plant foods rather than unhealthy ones.

Get Your Phytochemicals

The only place to get phytochemicals is through whole foods such as fruits, vegetables, beans, and whole grains. These essential nutrients directly impact your health. A few key phytochemicals might help prevent certain cancers, lower cholesterol, keep the gastrointestinal tract healthy, and protect various cells throughout the body. There are thousands of different forms available, but the most commonly known nutrients are terms that might be a little more familiar to you: flavonoids, antioxidants, and carotenoids.

How do you fill your diet with these amazing nutrients? Start by adding a rainbow of colors on your plate. The more colorful fruits and vegetables you consume, the higher your body's chances of receiving the nutrients it needs. There are many beautifully colored fruits and vegetables to choose from, including red tomatoes, blue blueberries, orange carrots, pink watermelon, pink grapefruit, green spinach, green kale, red strawberries, and red raspberries. To provide more benefits to your body, you should add lots of colors to your plate.

In addition to fruits and vegetables, phytonutrients can be found in whole-grain bread, whole-grain cereal, walnuts, sunflower seeds, peas, lentils, green tea, and black tea. If you consume bread and cereals, it is important to ensure that they are truly made from whole grains, not processed grains that could be stripped of the nutrients you assume you are obtaining by eating them.

Is Organic a Requirement?

Eating whole foods does not mean that they must be locally grown or even organic; that is a completely different topic. This does not mean that your whole foods cannot be organic; it is just not a prerequisite to qualify as whole or natural. Although, organic or locally grown food could provide you with the added benefit of eliminating harmful toxins and chemicals.

---

[1] Nuri Faruk Aykan, "Red Meat and Colorectal Cancer", *Oncology Reviews* 9, no. 1 (2015): 288,

Maximize Nutrients in Vegetables

Besides that, we eat food that tastes good to obtain the vital nutrients necessary for good health. When you consume food that has been modified, processed, or refined, the important nutrients are removed. This is even true for those foods that you consider healthy. For example, you might think you are doing your body well by eating spinach or broccoli, but if you do not eat it raw or prepare it properly, you are likely losing some of its nutrients, especially water-soluble elements. Vitamin B and C are two water-soluble vitamins found in both vegetables that are lost when cooked in water, whether boiled or steamed. Choosing to eat these vegetables raw is the best way to consume all vital nutrients. If you prefer them cooked, choose methods such as sautéing, stir-frying, or blanching, as each method is considered "quick-cooking" methods and avoids the risk of losing many nutrients.

Creating the Perfect Meals

Creating the perfect meals with the right plant-based whole foods does not have to be difficult. It is best to get creative to maximize the nutrients that you consume. Start with the basics, including whole-grain bread, whole-grain pasta, steel-cut oats, colorful fruits, and raw vegetables. Then, you can get creative:

- Add fruits and spices to your oatmeal
- Add flaxseed to your whole-grain cereal
- Make salad the main course for lunch or dinner and get creative
- Add your favorite vegetables to whole grain pasta or rice
- Make smoothies with as many fruits and vegetables as possible
- Add plant-based, natural nut butter to whole grain bread
- Eat fruit for dessert
- Add beans to lunch and dinner entrées
- Incorporate at least one fruit and vegetable at every meal

Protein is necessary for optimum health. According to the Protein Summit reports in AJCN, 16 percent is not excessive. In fact, the results indicate that Americans may consume too little protein rather than too much. Protein is more beneficial when spread out throughout the course of the day's meals and snacks, rather than filling up at supper, as many Americans do. The recommended daily protein intake is a MINIMUM of 0.1 g per kilogram of body weight for non-active individuals. Other evidence-based recommendations list a range of 1.2 g to 2.0 g per kilogram of body weight, based on an individual's level of physical activity.

Since the average American woman weighs about 170 pounds, and the average American man weighs about 197 pounds (according to multiple studies over the past three years).

An average-sized slightly "active" American woman should need AT LEAST 92.7 g of protein per day, according to the numbers ($170/2.2 = 77.3$ kg x $1.2 = 92.7$).

An average-sized, slightly "active" American male should need AT LEAST 107 g of protein per day, according to the numbers ($197/2.2 = 89.5$ kg x $1.2 = 107.4$).

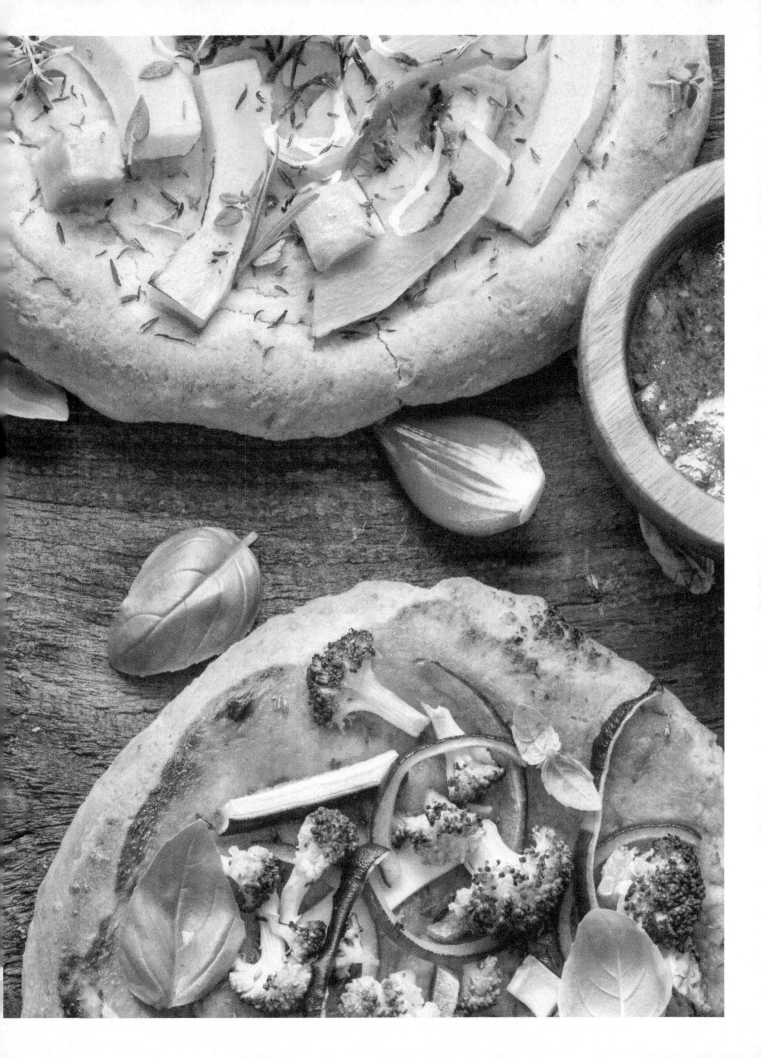

Chapter 2: Differences in Diet Between Plant-Based and Vegan Nutrition

Vegan Vs. Vegetarian Vs. Plant-Based

Vegan, vegetarian, and plant-based diets are very similar because they are based on vegetables, but they have certain distinctions.

Vegan

A vegan eats a plant-based diet — yet that is just a single portion of veganism. Aside from dairy, meat, fish, eggs, and nectar, vegans additionally maintain a strategic distance from animal-based added substances like gelatin and lanolin. Furthermore, vegans are convinced that the use of animal products should be banned, whether on their plates, makeup, cleaning items, clothes, or furniture.

Veganism is a way of life that looks to bar the use of animal products however much as could reasonably be expected. Going vegan is generally a choice one makes that is dependent on moral reasons, for example, a person can go vegan in the wake of finding out about the farming industry's poor treatment of animals.

This type of diet became popular recently, although many people practice it out of necessity, i.e., when they can't get a hold of eggs, dairy, meat, fish, etc. Some believe that veganism is more of a philosophy than a diet. It is based on the idea that the only way not to contribute to animal cruelty is to veer away from all animal products, i.e., meat, poultry, fish, shellfish, dairy, eggs, honey, leather, fur, wool, etc. This is a very healthy diet that needs to be carefully planned so you don't become nutrient-deficient as some of the essential nutrients are found only in animal-based foods.

Vegetarian

Officially, the vegetarian diet has existed since around 700 B.C. However, this is not true since human physiology clearly shows that we developed as omnivores (i.e., we ate whatever we could find). As collecting plants is easier and less risky than hunting, this is what people lived on for most of the year. Once technology improved and the first animals were domesticated, meat became easier to come by, and the human population exploded.

Today, those who adopt a vegetarian diet do it for many reasons, e.g., ethics, religion, environmentalism, health, etc. A vegetarian diet's essence is to refrain from poultry, beef, game, fish, shellfish, or any by-products of animals. However, while vegetarians do not eat meat, most use animal-derived products, e.g., fur, leather, or wool.

There are many vegetarian diets; the most common ones of which are:

- Lacto-Ovo vegetarian: The followers of this diet avoid all types of meat but consume dairy and eggs.
- Lacto vegetarian: They refrain from meat and eggs but use dairy.
- Ovo vegetarian: These are vegetarians who avoid meat and dairy but use eggs.
- Pescatarians: They do not eat meat or poultry but consume fish.
- Flexitarians: These are people who can be qualified as part-time vegetarians, i.e., they refrain from meat and fish from time to time.

Plant-Based

A plant-based diet consists mainly of plants but does not exclude meat and fish, although these are usually eaten only occasionally. There are many variations of this diet, and they are generally considered an extremely healthy way of eating.

However, a plant-based diet can also be very unhealthy if it is based on plant-based foods and includes refined grains and plant-based junk foods, e.g., sugary beverages, sweets, high-starch foods, etc. So, a plant-based diet is only healthy if it is based on whole grains, healthy fats, and healthy protein.

Besides, it's even more important to focus on high-quality foods on a plant-only diet (this is different from a plant-based diet).

Overall, eating a plant-based diet with well-being as your inspiration is an extraordinary thing. Not only can eating, for the most part, plants help forestall and invert sickness, but it also helps in weight loss and added wellbeing. You will also appreciate the positive reactions of reducing your ecological footprint as you will hurt fewer animals.

What to Eat and What to Avoid

Most people prefer to eat animal-based products for every meal. The focus of the plant-based diet plan is to make plant-based foods the primary food source. Consume animal-based foods in smaller quantities if you have a craving for them. Instead of making the animal-based foods the central part of the dish, use these foods, like seafood, meat, eggs, poultry, and dairy, as a side dish. Listed below are plant-based foods to make your choices easier:

- Fruits: Bananas, pears, berries, citrus fruits, pineapples, peach, etc.
- Veggies: Peppers, broccoli, spinach, asparagus, tomatoes, kale, carrots, cauliflower, etc.
- Whole Grains: Rolled oats, farro, barley, quinoa, brown rice pasta, brown rice, etc.
- Starchy Veggies: Potatoes, butternut squash, sweet potatoes, etc.
- Legumes: Peas, peanuts, black beans, chickpeas, lentils, etc.
- Plant-Based Milk (Unsweetened): Almond milk, cashew milk, coconut milk, etc.
- Condiments: Mustard, lemon juice, soy sauce, salsa, nutritional yeast, vinegar, etc.
- Nuts, Nut Butter, and Seeds: Pumpkin seeds, sunflower seeds, tahini, cashews, almonds, macadamia nuts, natural peanut butter (sugar-free), etc.
- Pork and Beef: If possible, select pasture-raised or grass-fed.
- Dairy Products: If possible, choose organic dairy products from pasture-raised animals.
- Seafood: If possible, pick wild-caught from sustainable fisheries.

As for foods, to avoid or limit on the plant-based diet plan, the primary focus of a plant-based diet plan is to avoid as much artificially produced food as possible and add natural foods to your plate. Heavily processed foods are strictly prohibited in a plant-based diet plan. So, you must choose fresh foods when you are purchasing grocery items. Select the packaged food with the least amount of ingredients if you need to buy them. The foods that need to be avoided on a plant-based diet plan include added sugars and sweets like candy, soda, sugary cereals, pastries, sweet tea, table sugar, juice, cookies, etc. The foods that must be restricted for a plant-based diet plan, even if you include healthy animal-based products in your diet, are game, pork, sheep, beef, dairy, seafood, eggs, and poultry.

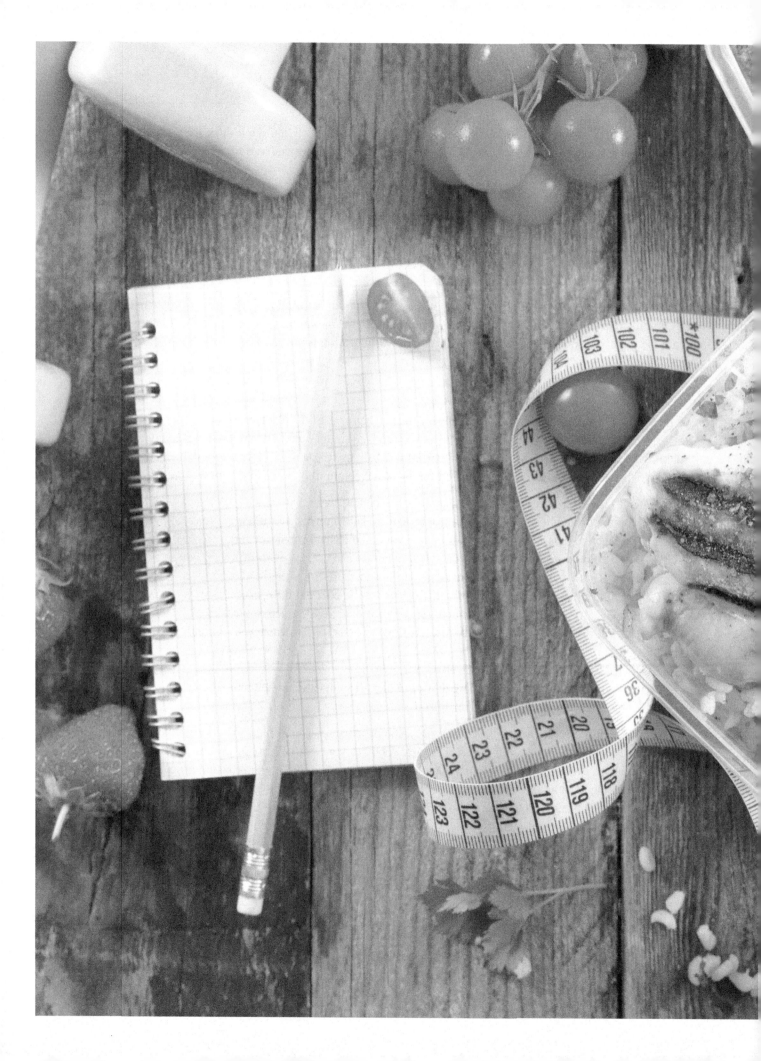

Chapter 3: Plant-Based Basic Guidelines

Getting started on whole plant-based diets is sometimes tricky and not as easy as we think. There is always a misconception among people. We think we are suddenly diet experts who automatically become super healthy when switching to plant-based diets. This is a big fallacy that causes most people who wish to go plant-based to lose interest early. It is also important to understand that thousands of plant-based junk foods, such as frozen veggie pizza and non-dairy ice cream, are out there in the market, which may be harmful to your health if you consistently consume them.

When consuming or trying to live a plant-based lifestyle, plant-based snacks can be a motivation source when taken in moderation and small bits.

Like the popular maxim that says, "Every big idea started small." Going plant-based might require you to take a step at a time – in doing this, let's look at how we can get started on whole plant-based recipes.

Determine What Plant-Based Meal Means to You

The first step in starting with these whole food plant-based diets is deciding how to structure your plant-based diet. This decision will help you in your transition from your current diet outlook. This step is personal and varies from one person to another. You might decide not to tolerate any form of animal-based food or products. At the same time, another person may occasionally put up bits by bits of meat; all this depends on personal preference on how the plant-based lifestyle will look. Don't allow any other person's lifestyle to put you down or make you feel that you are not doing it well. The only thing consistent in this lifestyle is that plant-based meals are the great majority of your meals.

Know What You Are Eating

After you have gone past the decision-making stage on how your plant-based dieting and lifestyle will look, the next stage will be to understand the different plant-based diets and foods in the market. Many plant-based diets and meals exist in the market, especially packaged foods containing some elements of animal products. As an individual transitioning to a whole plant-based lifestyle, it is important to nurture a habit of reading labels when shopping. It is necessary to keep an eye on the ingredient labels to avoid foods that might potentially impact your health in the long run.

Look-Out for an Overhaul Version of Your Choice Diets

One of the hardest parts of going plant-based is leaving behind all your favorite meals. But it doesn't have to be so. There is usually a middle point when you are going fully plant-based in your diets. Consider some non-plant-based foods that you used to love based on their flavor, texture, and so on, then look for an alternative within the whole plant-based recipe that can fill in those gaps and cravings. For example, lentils can be a great source of alternative for meatloaf and Bolognese when going fully plant-based.

Have A Support Network

Building a support network when you are starting up a plant-based lifestyle is very important. This is important since commencing a new habit can be tough when done alone. Surround yourself with friends and families that share the same belief system and lifestyle in dieting and are willing to live this lifestyle with you. With supportive friends and relatives around, they can help you stay focused and motivated since they are there to provide emotional support. These support systems can share new plant-based recipes and plant-based options for you. You can also become part of some support system online or with the local plant-based groups within your locality.

First Steps to Start the Diet

Be Mentally and Psychologically Ready

Eating food is a daily routine that human beings are supposed to undergo. The nature of substances and foods we consume daily can result in a lifetime consumption habit if not regulated. Once habits form, it is difficult to break them. People surrounding us can also contribute to influencing your habits or hinder transformation. So, before jumping into a new lifestyle, you need to properly think about it. It will help you avoid making empty promises to yourself. After you have already thought of your move to plant-based dieting, look into the obstacles that will prevent you either psychologically or mentally in your transformation journey. With the knowledge of the distractions, your chances of successfully getting into the diet are high.

Drink More Water

Consumption of water is vital. Water helps in maintaining brain health and other body operations. So, you need to replace the water that is used in the process. You should always be hydrated. The doctor here recommends taking in spring water since they are normally in an alkaline state. Tap water is often contaminated with chemicals such as chloride compounds and other chemicals.

According to doctors, one should drink a gallon of spring water on a minimum daily. Avoid taking water-containing softeners. Water from reverse osmosis systems should be avoided too. The work of the water is to help in nutrient absorption and organ and joint cushioning. Remember that existing health organizations do recommend the intake of a gallon of water as well. You should also make a habit/culture of drinking water.

Include Extra Whole Meals to Your Diet

Whole foods range from fruits that you like to fresh fish fillets. You should distance yourself from consuming foods that are kept in packages as they are addictive. Restraining from these foods will greatly assist you as you advance through a plant-based diet.

Work hard in completely substituting processed meals with whole foods as a lot of processed foods contain sugars that are enhanced. These sugars are considered addictive as they can trigger cravings for these types of food.

Read the Ingredient Labels

Avoiding other types of food can be difficult most times. So, you can resort to reading the labels of the products to know what they contain. It keeps you in the know-how of what you take into your body. The habit also assists in directing you in what to change from the foods you eat. It will also assist you once you have fully embraced the diet. In this stage, you will be knowledgeable of whatever you consume.

One of the most useful devices when shopping for meal preparation is the freezer, but you must keep some things in mind to make your life easier. You must clean out your freezer regularly, and you must store your food at room temperature or in the refrigerator before freezing. This is so that your food is not hot when you put it in – hot food thaws the ice and food around it which can cause spoilage.

Keeping the freezer full is more economical, and the air will be kept cold more easily. However, don't overload it as that can cause little to no air circulation. Be careful not to keep the door open for long when taking food in and out, as the food inside will start to defrost and go bad.

Chapter 4: 28-Day Meal Plan

To get the complete plant-based diet experience, stick to this meal plan for the next month. It arranges breakfast, lunch, snack, dinner, and dessert every day, based on recipes and plant-based eating criteria. These meals are intended for four people. Divide the ingredients by 2 if you have 2 family members, and multiply by 1.5 if you have 6 family members.

For one individual, the plan is based on 1800/2,000 calories per day, and 25 grams of sugar per day. Feel free to add small snacks and juices/smoothies as you please, and don't forget to drink 3 liters of water per day at least. Enjoy!

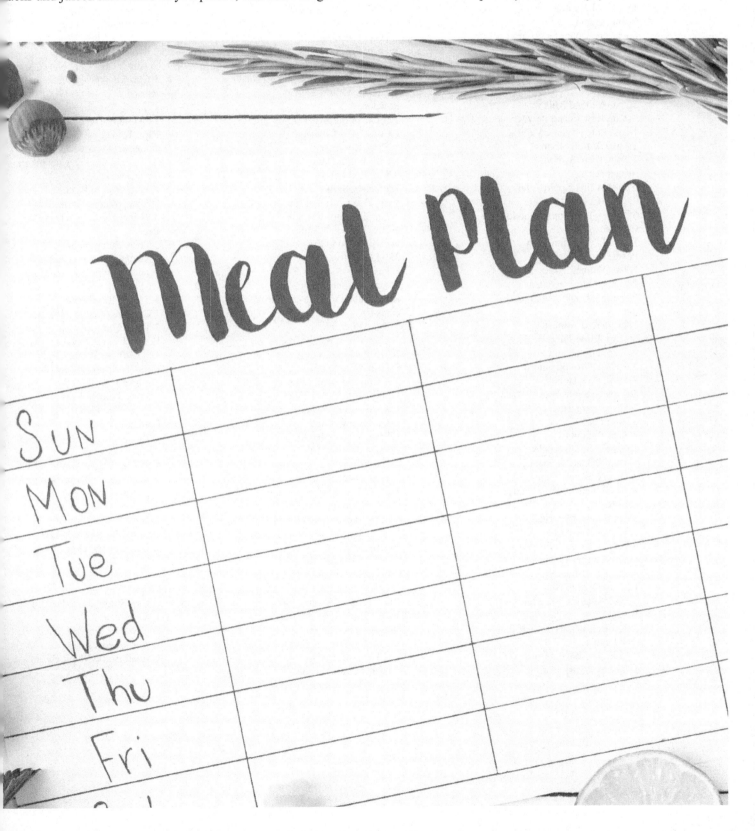

1. Week 1 Shopping List

- 1.75 Cups Rolled Oats
- 3 ½ Cups Porridge Oats
- ⅓ Cup Cocoa Powder
- 1 Cup Dates
- 1 Cup Coconut Flakes, Unsweetened
- 1 Cup All-Natural Smooth Peanut Butter
- 6 Frozen Bananas + 3 Large Bananas
- ¼ Cup Nuts Seeds
- 4 Avocados + 6 Ripe Hass Avocados
- 30 oz. Almond Milk
- ½ Cup Raw Cacao Powder
- 1 tsp.. Pure Organic Vanilla + 1 Tbsp. Vanilla Extract
- 2 To 4 Tbsp. Swerve Sweetener
- 0.76 lb. Cups Apple Cider
- 0.78 lb. Coconut Yogurt
- 6 Tbsp. +1.75 Cups Almonds, Crushed
- 1 Small Pack Cinnamon Powder
- ½ tsp. Nutmeg
- 2 Canned Unsweetened Pineapple Chunks or Fresh 16 oz.
- 2 Large Red Apples
- 8 Tbsp. Lime Juice
- 9 Tbsp. Lemon Juice
- 3½ Tbsp. Ground Ginger
- 9 Tbsp. Raw Honey
- 2 Cups Green Grapes
- 2 Tbsp. Margarine
- 6 Bosc Pears,
- ½ Cup Walnuts
- 1 Granny Smith Apple
- ¼ Cup Pickled Jalapenos
- 2 Tbsp. Cayenne Pepper
- 4 oz. Grated Vegan Cheddar Cheese
- 3 tsp. Smoked Paprika
- 1.5 Tbsp. Mustard Powder
- 6 Tbsp. Flax Seed Powder
- 6.5 oz. Crumbled Tofu
- 8 oz. Tofu Cheese
- 12.5 oz. Vegan Butter
- 8.5 lb. Potatoes, Sliced Into Wedges
- 2 Red Bell Pepper + 1 Green Bell Pepper
- 0.15 lb. Fresh Cilantro
- 3 Garlics + 1 tsp. Garlic Powder
- 2 Slices Vegan Bacon
- 1 Shallot
- 24 oz. Green Beans
- 2 tsp. Vinegar
- 1 lb. Turnips, Sliced Into Cubes
- 12 oz. Vegan Parmesan Cheese
- 1 Tbsp. Fresh Thyme,
- 1 Tbsp. Fresh Chives, Chopped
- 255 ml. Coconut Oil
- 3.5 Tbsp. Yellow Curry Powder
- 1 tsp. Onion Powder
- 2 Cups Napa Cabbage
- 1 Tbsp. Rosemary
- 1.5 lb. White Onion
- 0.5 lb. Red Onion
- 1.5 Celery Stalks
- 1 tsp. Red Chili Flakes
- ½ Cup Popcorn Kernels
- 4 Tbsp. Coconut Sugar
- ¼ Cup Walnut Oil
- 250 l.ml. Olive Oil
- 5 Tbsp. Soy Sauce
- 26 oz. Tempeh Bacon, Homemade Or Store-Bought 2 Cups Rice Broccoli
- 5 Tbsp. Plain Flour
- ½ Cup Mixed Salad Greens
- 10-15 Radishes, Large
- 8 Tbsp. Chia Seeds
- 2 ½ Cups Almond Flour
- 1 Tbsp. Nutritional Yeast
- 1 tsp. Baking Powder
- ¾ Cup Brown Rice
- 1 Tbsp. Vegetable Oil
- 24 oz. Coconut Milk
- 4 Cod Fillets
- 1 lb. Brussels Sprouts, Trimmed And Sliced In Half
- ¼ Cup Coconut Water
- 8 Cups Cauliflower Florets
- 1.5 Cup Parsley
- 3 Cups Arugula
- 0.75 Cup Black Olives + ½ Cup Green Olives
- ¼ Cup Feta, Crumbled
- 2 tsp. Toasted Sesame Oil
- 30 oz. Canned White Bean, Drained And Rinsed
- ½ Cup Cashew Cream
- 1 ½ Tbsp. Miso Paste
- 1 Tbsp. Sesame Seeds
- 4 Slices Rye Bread, Toasted
- 1/2 Teaspoon Turmeric
- 1.5 Teaspoon Cumin
- ½ Cup Vegan Guacamole, For Serving
- 1 ½ Cup Pico De Gallo
- 18 oz. Blueberries
- 1 ½ tsp. Stevia Powder
- ¼ Cup Pecans, Chopped
- 1 ½ Cups Whole Wheat Flour
- 2 tsp. Baking Soda
- ½ Cup Vegan Chocolate Chips
- 1 Cup Chickpeas, Drained And Rinsed
- 1 Small Tomato, Sliced + ½ Cup Grape Tomatoes +2 Large Ripe Tomatoes +3 Ripe Roma Tomatoes
- 2 Medium English Cucumbers
- 7 Carrots, Diced
- 4 Tbsp. Tahini Paste
- 8 Slices Whole-Grain Bread
- 8 (7-Inch) Whole-Wheat Pita Bread
- 1 Tbsp. Pumpkin Seeds
- 1 Mango + ½ Cup Chopped Mango Chutney, Homemade Or Store-Bought
- 1.5 Cups Raspberries
- 1 Cup Chopped Fresh Kale
- 2 Tbsp. Flaxseeds
- ½ Cup Unsweetened Soy Milk
- 12 (10-Inch) Whole-Grain Flour Tortillas Or Lavash Flatbread
- 8 Large Lettuce Leaves
- 3 Cups Shredded Romaine Lettuce
- 16 Small Boston Or Other Soft Lettuce Leaves
- 4.83 Cup Vegan Mayonnaise, Homemade Or Store-Bought
- 4 tsp. Dijon Mustard
- 3 ½ Cups Whole-Wheat Flour
- 1 Cup Marinara Sauce
- 2 Large Zucchinis, Sliced
- ½ Cup Chopped Spinach
- 1 Jicama Bulb
- ½ Cup Dairy-Free Chocolate Chips
- ½ Cup Strawberries Halved
- 1 Watermelon
- ½ Cup Pomegranate Seeds
- ½ Cup Cherries
- 1 Small Bottle Maple Syrup

2. Week 1 Meal Plan

DAY 1	
BreakFast	High Protein Toast - no.9. - pg.24
Snack a.m	Avocado and Tempeh Bacon Wraps - no.19. - pg.28
Lunch	Cauliflower Salad - no.106. - pg.66
Snack p.m	Watermelon Pizza - no.31. - pg.33
Dinner	Cheesy Potato Casserole - no.107. - pg.67
Dessert	Almond Pulp Cookies - no.185. - pg.100

Tot. Nut. *Kcal, 1996*
Protein, 78.7g
Carbs, 111g
Fat, 109.7g

DAY 2	
BreakFast	Sweet Potato Breakfast Hash - no.17. - pg.27
Snack a.m	Curried Tofu "Egg Salad" Pitas - no.21. - pg.29
Lunch	Coconut Brussels sprouts - no.108. - pg.67
Snack p.m	Tamari Toasted Almonds - no.29. - pg.32
Dinner	Rosemary Sweet Potato Medallions - no.109. - pg.67
Dessert	Sautéed Pears - no.186. - pg.100

Tot. Nut. *Kcal, 1720*
Protein, 78g
Carbs, 168g
Fat, 73g

DAY 3	
BreakFast	Chocolate Chip Banana Pancake - no.8. - pg.24
Snack a.m	Grilled Zucchini and Spinach Pizza - no.23. - pg.30
Lunch	Cod Stew with Rice & Sweet Potatoes - no.110. - pg.68
Snack p.m	Honey-Almond Popcorn - no.24. - pg.30
Dinner	Curried Tofu with Buttery Cabbage - no.111. - pg.68
Dessert	Fruit Skewers - no.187. - pg.101

Tot. Nut. *Kcal, 1994.4*
Protein, 80g
Carbs, 215.8g
Fat, 86.2g

DAY 4	
BreakFast	Hummus Carrot Sandwich - no.10. - pg.24
Snack a.m	Jicama and Guacamole - no.25. - pg.31
Lunch	Curry Mushroom Pie - no.112. - pg.69
Snack p.m	Grilled Zucchini and Spinach Pizza - no.23. - pg.30
Dinner	Garlic Mashed Potatoes & Turnips - no.113. - pg.69
Dessert	Apple Almond Slush - no.188. - pg.101

Tot. Nut. *Kcal, 1980*
Protein, 65.2g
Carbs, 183.7g
Fat, 131.9g

DAY 5	
BreakFast	Overnight Oats - no.15. - pg.26
Snack a.m	Peanut Butter Chip Cookies - no.27. - pg.31
Lunch	Pecan & Blueberry Crumble - no.115. - pg.70
Snack p.m	Jicama and Guacamole - no.25. - pg.31
Dinner	Green Beans with vegan Bacon - no.114. - pg.70
Dessert	Avocado Pudding - no.189. - pg.101

Tot. Nut. *Kcal, 1909*
Protein, 82g
Carbs, 93.7g
Fat, 127.4g

DAY 6	
BreakFast	Avocado Toast with White Beans - no.1. - pg.21
Snack a.m	Garden Salad Wraps - no.22. - pg.29
Lunch	Radish Chips - no.116. - pg.70
Snack p.m	Avocado and Tempeh Bacon Wraps - no.19. - pg.28
Dinner	Roasted Sweet Potatoes... - no.117. - pg.71
Dessert	Banana Ice Cream - no.190. - pg.102

Tot. Nut. *Kcal, 1937*
Protein, 69.8g
Carbs, 104g
Fat, 117.2g

DAY 7	
BreakFast	Super Smoothie - no.18. - pg.27
Snack a.m	Watermelon Pizza - no.31. - pg.33
Lunch	Smoked Tempeh with Broccoli Fritters - no.118. - pg.71
Snack p.m	Curried Tofu "Egg Salad" Pitas - no.21. - pg.29
Dinner	Spicy Cheesy Tofu Balls - no.119. - pg.72
Dessert	Chocolate Peanut Butter Energy Bites - no.191. - pg.102

Tot. Nut. *Kcal, 1983*
Protein, 68.4g
Carbs, 125g
Fat, 145g

3. Week 2 Shopping List

- 26 oz. Shredded Coconut
- 3 Cans Coconut Milk, Unsweetened- Full Fat
- 6 oz. Coconut Sugar
- 8 fl. oz. Coconut Oil
- 1 Tbsp. Tapioca Starch
- 1 Small Bottle Vanilla Extract
- 1 Green Tea Bag
- 26 oz. Fresh Blueberries
- 1 Pear, Peeled, Cored, And Diced
- 24 fl. oz. Almond Milk
- 6.75 oz. Sugar-Free Chocolate Chips
- 2 tsp. Stevia
- 15 oz. Pecans, Chopped
- 4.5 oz. Cranberries
- ¼ Cup Raspberries
- 0.3 lb. Fresh Ginger, Finely Grated
- 4 Fresh Lemons, Juiced
- 1.2 lb. Almond Flour
- 0.5 lb. Coconut Flour
- 1 tsp. Baking Soda
- 1 Pack Sea Salt
- 1 Cup Nut Butter
- 1 Cup Coconut Palm Sugar
- 6.75 oz. Organic Raisins
- 1 Large & 1 Medium Ripe Avocado
- 3 Tbsp. Raw Cacao Powder
- 1 Small Bottle Coconut Nectar or Agave
- 1 Pack of Cinnamon Powder
- 1 Cup Frozen Strawberries
- 1 Apple
- 3.5 oz. Hemp Seeds
- 5 Limes, Juiced
- 20 fl oz. Light Mayonnaise
- 5 Scallions
- 4 Cups Mixed Salad Greens
- 2.5 Tbsp. White Miso
- 2 Tbsp. Chopped Fresh Dill
- 6.75 oz. Crumbled Tempeh
- 5 Grape Tomatoes +3 Ripe Roma Tomatoes
- 28 oz. Canned Crushed Tomatoes +10 oz. Cherry Tomatoes
- ½ Cup Dry Quinoa +1 Cup Cooked Quinoa
- ½ Cup Dry Navy Beans
- 3 Cans (15 oz. Each) Chickpeas
- 0.75 Cup Extra-Virgin Olive Oil
- 1 Small Pack Paprika Powder

- 1 Tbsp. Cayenne
- 1 Tbsp. Chili Powder
- 1.2 lb. Spinach, Fresh or Frozen
- 1 Purple Onion + 3 Onion + 1 Red Onion
- 4 tsp. Onion Powder
- 3.2 lb. Potatoes
- 2 Tbsp. Fresh Chives
- 3 (15 oz.) Canned White Beans
- 1 Bottle Olive Oil
- 2 Heads Garlic + 3 tsp. Garlic Powder
- 1 Large Eggplant
- 6 Lavash Wraps or Large Pita Bread
- 8 oz. Creamy Traditional Hummus
- 7 oz. Vegan Feta Cheese, Crumbled or Chopped
- 6 fl. oz. Honey
- 1-2 tsp. Ground Cumin
- 2 tsp. Chili Flakes
- 8 oz. Okra
- 10 oz. Vegan Butter
- 1 Head of Baby Bok Choy, Quartered Lengthwise
- 8 oz. Sliced Mushrooms
- 3 lb. Extra-Firm Tofu
- 8 oz. Tofu Cheese
- 2 Tbsp. Plain Vinegar
- 2.5 Tbsp. Sesame Oil
- Wasabi Paste, to Taste
- Cooked White or Brown Rice (½ Cup Per Person)
- 2 Cups of Rice Broccoli
- 4 lb. Large Acorn Squash
- 8 fl. oz. Vegetable Stock
- 1 lb. Medjool Dates
- 6.75 oz. Walnuts
- 2 tsp. Ground Turmeric
- 2 Tbsp. Cocoa Powder, Unsweetened
- ½ Cup Panko Breadcrumbs
- 1½ Cups Cold Green Pea Risotto
- 3 ½ Cups Whole-Wheat Flour
- 1 tsp. Yeast
- 1 Cup Red Pizza Sauce
- ¼ Cup Grated Plant-Based Parmesan Cheese
- 10 oz. Raw Whole Almonds
- 6.75 oz. Roasted Almonds
- 4 Bunches Kale
- 4 Tbsp. Avocado Oil
- 10 oz. Cup Jarred Roasted Peppers

- 1 tsp. Italian Seasoning
- 1/2 Cup Shredded Broccoli Florets
- 1/2 Cup Shredded Carrots
- 2 Teaspoon Parsley
- 1/2 Cup Bread Crumbs, Gluten-Free
- 2 Flax Eggs
- 4 Cups Frozen Mixed Berries
- 4 Small Frozen Bananas + 1 Fresh
- 4 Scoops of Vanilla Protein Powder
- 6 oz. Chia Seeds
- ½ Cup Granola
- 1 ½ Rolled Oats
- ½ Cup Non-Dairy Milk
- ½ Cup Sun-Butter
- ½ Cup Apple Sauce
- 1 Cup Alfalfa Sprouts
- 2 Fresh Mangoes, Diced
- Maple Syrup
- ¼ Cup Pickled Jalapenos
- 4 oz. Grated Vegan Cheddar Cheese
- 1 Tbsp. Mustard Powder
- 1 Tbsp. Flax Seed Powder
- 1 Red Bell Pepper
- ¼ Cup Fresh Cilantro
- 2 Slices of Vegan Bacon
- 1 Shallot
- 24 oz. Green Beans
- 1 Cup Popcorn Kernels
- ½ Cup Walnut Oil
- 10-15 Radishes, Large
- ½ Cup Cashew Cream
- 1 Tbsp. Sesame Seeds
- 4 Slices Rye Bread, Toasted
- 1 Tbsp. Soy Sauce
- ¼ Cup Apple Cider Vinegar
- 1 tsp. Yellow or Spicy Brown Mustard
- 3 Cups Shredded Romaine Lettuce
- 1 Large Carrot, Shredded
- 1 Medium English Cucumber
- ¼ Cup Sliced Pitted Green Olives
- 4 (10-Inch) Whole-Grain Flour Tortillas
- 4 Tbsp. Flax Seed Powder
- 1 Tbsp. Soy Sauce
- 10 oz. Tempeh Slices
- 3 Tbsp. Plain Flour
- ½ Cup Mixed Salad Greens
- 4 Tbsp. Tamari

4. Week 2 Meal Plan

DAY 8	
BreakFast	Mango Agua Fresca - no.13. - pg.25
Snack a.m	Chickpea Avocado Pizza - no.20. - pg.28
Lunch	Tofu Cabbage Stir-Fry - no.120. - pg.72
Snack p.m	Turmeric Snack Bites - no.30. - pg.32
Dinner	Simple Baked Okra - no.121. - pg.73
Dessert	Cinnamon Berry Slush - no.192. - pg.102

Tot. Nut.	Kcal, 1955	Protein, 76g
		Carbs, 208g
		Fat, 107g

DAY 9	
BreakFast	Banana and Chai Chia Smoothie... - no.2. - pg.21
Snack a.m	Tamari Toasted Almonds - no.29. - pg.32
Lunch	Green Beans with vegan Bacon - no.114. - pg.70
Snack p.m	White Bean Stuffed Squash - no.32. - pg.33
Dinner	Chickpea and Spinach Salad... - no.124. - pg.75
Dessert	Cocoa Avocado Ice Cream - no.193. - pg.103

Tot. Nut.	Kcal, 1868	Protein, 56g
		Carbs, 140g
		Fat, 128.8g

DAY 10	
BreakFast	Sun-Butter Baked Oatmeal Cups - no.16. - pg.27
Snack a.m	Honey-Almond Popcorn - no.24. - pg.30
Lunch	Pecan & Blueberry Crumble - no.115. - pg.70
Snack p.m	Garden Salad Wraps - no.22. - pg.29
Dinner	Grilled Veggie and Hummus Wrap - no.129. - pg.77
Dessert	Coconut Raisins Cookies - no.194. - pg.103

Tot. Nut.	Kcal, 1980	Protein, 74g
		Carbs, 118g
		Fat, 125g

DAY 11	
BreakFast	Berries and Banana Smoothie Bowl - no.3. - pg.22
Snack a.m	Kale Bowls - no.26. - pg.31
Lunch	Radish Chips - no.116. - pg.70
Snack p.m	Honey-Almond Popcorn - no.24. - pg.30
Dinner	Greek Style Beans - no.128. - pg.77
Dessert	Cranberry Refresher - no.195. - pg.104

Tot. Nut.	Kcal, 1824	Protein, 52.8g
		Carbs, 128g
		Fat, 79g

DAY 12	
BreakFast	Hummus Carrot Sandwich... - no.10. - pg.24
Snack a.m	Risotto Bites - no.28. - pg.32
Lunch	Roasted Sweet Potatoes - no.117. - pg.71
Snack p.m	Kale Bowls - no.26. - pg.31
Dinner	Mashed Potatoes with Spinach - no.133. - pg.79
Dessert	Crunchy Bars - no.196. - pg.104

Tot. Nut.	Kcal, 1637	Protein, 85g
		Carbs, 196g
		Fat, 72g

DAY 13	
BreakFast	Broccoli and Quinoa Breakfast Patties - no.4. - pg.22
Snack a.m	Turmeric Snack Bites - no.30. - pg.32
Lunch	Smoked Tempeh with Broccoli F... - no.118. - pg.71
Snack p.m	Risotto Bites - no.28. - pg.32
Dinner	Roasted Almond Protein Salad - no.134. - pg.79
Dessert	Green Tea Blueberry Shake - no.197. - pg.104

Tot. Nut.	Kcal, 1899	Protein, 57.9g
		Carbs, 139.7g
		Fat, 82g

DAY 14	
BreakFast	High Protein Toast... - no.9. - pg.24
Snack a.m	White Bean Stuffed Squash... - no.32. - pg.33
Lunch	Spicy Cheesy Tofu Balls - no.119. - pg.72
Snack p.m	Tamari Toasted Almonds - no.29. - pg.32
Dinner	Tempeh "Chicken" Salad - no.143. - pg.83
Dessert	Homemade Coconut Ice Cream - no.0 - pg.104

Tot. Nut.	Kcal, 1787	Protein, 75g
		Carbs, 122.6g
		Fat, 118.2g

5. Week 3 Shopping List

- 1.6 lb. Almond Flour
- 11 fl. oz. Nut Butter
- ½ Cup Erythritol
- 1.2 lb. Strawberries
- 1 Cup Kiwis
- 8 oz. Blueberries
- 3 oz. Raspberries
- 5 oz. Blackberries
- 1 Cup Pineapple Chunks
- 2 tsp. Lime Zest
- 4 Limes, Juiced
- 8 fl. oz. Coconut Oil
- 2 Scoops Of Vanilla Protein
- Stevia, To Taste
- 1 Small Pack Cinnamon
- 2 oz. Almond Butter
- ¼ Cup Swerve
- 13 fl. oz. Peanut Butter
- 1 tsp. Lemon Zest
- 16 fl. oz. Coconut Cream
- 4.5 oz. Macadamia Nuts
- 9 oz. Dates
- 8 fl. oz. Maple Syrup
- 5 Lemons, Juiced
- 9 oz. Cashews
- 12 fl. oz. Coconut Milk, Unsweetened
- 1 Fresh Mango
- 3.2 lb. Whole-Wheat Flour
- 8 (10-Inch) Soft Flour Tortillas Or Lavash Flatbread
- 1 lb. Flaxseed Powder
- ¼ Cup Plant Butter, Cold, And Crumbled
- 10 oz. Cashew Cream
- 1 lb. Pure Date Sugar Or Coconut Sugar
- 1 Cup Mixed Frozen Berries
- 0.5 lb. Organic Buckwheat Noodles
- 3 Heads Garlic
- 8 Onions +1 Medium White Onion +1 Medium Red Onion
- 1 Laminated Leek
- 8 Carrots
- 1.2 lb. Laminated Mushrooms
- 3 Celeries
- ½ Red Pepper
- ½ Green Pepper
- 1 Fresh Ginger
- 1 Strip Wakame Seaweed
- 16 fl oz. Olive Oil
- 5 fl. oz. Soy Sauce
- 2 bunches Parsley
- 0.5 lb. Textured Vegetable Protein, Chunks
- ½ Cup Split Red Lentils
- 1 Cup Sliced Parsnip
- 35 fl. oz. Vegetable Stock
- 1 Cup Rutabaga
- 2 Bay Leaves

- 1 lb. Ground Black Pepper & Salt
- 0.8 oz. Thyme
- 2 tsp. Marmite
- 2 oz. Rosemary
- ¼ tsp. Marjoram
- 1 Cup Anasazi Beans
- 2.5 lb. Vegetable Broth
- 1 Bay Laurel
- 2 Bell Peppers
- 1 Green Chili Pepper
- 1 Tbsp. Cayenne Pepper
- 1 Small Packet Paprika Powder
- 3 Cans (15 oz. Each) Chickpeas
- 12 Cherry Tomatoes
- 5 oz. Sliced Grape Tomatoes
- 4 Ripe Roma Tomatoes
- A Handful Of String Beans
- 1 Apple
- 5 oz. Raisins
- A Handful Of Fresh Mint
- 2 Oranges
- 6 oz. Red Beans
- 3 oz. Unsweetened Cocoa Powder
- 4 Bananas
- 5 Frozen Bananas
- 1 tsp. Maca Powder
- 4 fl. oz. Unsweetened Soy Milk
- 12 oz. Rolled Oats
- 50 oz. Fresh Spinach
- 4 Scoops Of Chocolate Protein Powder
- 6 oz. Vegan Dark Chocolate
- 1 tsp. Peppermint Extract, Unsweetened
- 4 fl. oz. Honey
- 45 fl. oz. Almond Milk, Unsweetened
- 1 Cup Hazelnuts, Unsalted, Roasted
- 10.6 fl. oz. Vegan Mayonnaise, Homemade Or Store-Bought
- 2 Scallions
- 4 Cups Mixed Salad Greens
- 1 oz. White Miso
- 2 Tbsp. Chopped Fresh Dill
- 1 ½ Cups Crumbled Tempeh
- 8 oz. Tempeh Bacon, Homemade Or Store-Bought
- 1 Large Eggplant
- 6 Lavash Wraps or Large Pita Bread
- 1 Cup Creamy Traditional Hummus
- 7 oz. Vegan Feta Cheese, Crumbled Or Chopped
- 3 tsp. Ground Cumin
- 1 tsp. Chili Flakes
- 8 oz. Okra
- 2 lb. Large Acorn Squash
- 25 oz. Can White Beans

- 5 oz. Walnuts
- Ground Turmeric
- ½ Cup Shredded Coconut, Unsweetened
- ½ Cup Panko Breadcrumbs
- 1½ Cups Cold Green Pea Risotto
- 4.5 oz. Almonds
- 2 Bunches Kale
- 2 fl. oz. Avocado Oil
- ⅔ Cup Jarred Roasted Peppers
- 1 tsp. Italian Seasoning
- ¼ tsp. Chili Powder
- 8 fl. oz. Red Pizza Sauce
- 5 Medium Avocados
- 10 fl. oz. Vegan Parmesan Cheese
- ¼ Cup Pickled Jalapenos
- 4 oz. Grated Vegan Cheddar Cheese
- 4 Tbsp. Dijon Mustard
- 3.2 lb. Crumbled Tofu
- 2 fl. oz. Vegan Butter
- 6 lb. Potatoes
- 1 Red Bell Pepper
- 6 oz. Fresh Cilantro
- 1 lb. Turnips
- 1 Tbsp. Fresh Chives
- 1 tsp. Garlic Powder
- 2 tsp. Toasted Sesame Oil
- 1 Tbsp. Sesame Seeds
- 4 Slices Rye Bread, Toasted
- ½ Cup Vegan Guacamole
- 1 ½ Cup Pico De Gallo
- 3 tsp. Baking Soda
- 7 oz. Vegan Chocolate Chips
- 2 tsp. Tahini Paste
- 4 Slices Whole-Grain Bread, Toasted
- 8 Large Lettuce Leaves
- ¼ Cup Chopped Mango Chutney, Homemade Or Store-Bought
- 1 Tbsp. Hot Or Mild Curry Powder
- 8 Small Boston Or Other Soft Lettuce Leaves
- 4 (7-Inch) Whole-Wheat Pita Bread, Halved
- 1 Tbsp. Yeast
- 1 Cup Marinara Sauce
- 2 Large Zucchinis
- ¼ Cup Black Olives
- ¼ Cup Green Olives
- 1 Jicama Bulb
- ¼ Cup Apple Cider Vinegar
- 1 Medium English Cucumber
- 1 Watermelon
- 1 Cup Coconut Yogurt
- ½ Cup Pomegranate Seeds
- ½ Cup Cherries
- 2 Tbsp. Tamari Or Soy Sauce

6. Week 3 Meal Plan

DAY 15	
BreakFast	Chocolate Chip Banana Pancake - no.8. - pg.24
Snack a.m	Jicama and Guacamole - no.25. - pg.31
Lunch	Stewed Kidney Bean - no.78. - pg.53
Snack p.m	Avocado and Tempeh Bacon Wraps - no.19. - pg.28
Dinner	Vegetarian Irish Stew - no.82. - pg.54
Dessert	Mango Coconut Cheesecake - no.0 - pg.105

Tot. Nut.	Kcal, 1652	Protein, 75g
		Carbs, 103g
		Fat, 77g

DAY 16	
BreakFast	High Protein Toast - no.9. - pg.24
Snack a.m	Tamari Toasted Almonds - no.29. - pg.32
Lunch	Rosemary Sweet Potato Medallions - no.109. - pg.67
Snack p.m	White Bean Stuffed Squash - no.32. - pg.33
Dinner	Soup of Noodles with Vegetables - no.76. - pg.52
Dessert	Mini Berry Tarts - no.0 - pg.105

Tot. Nut.	Kcal, 1876	Protein, 77g
		Carbs, 139g
		Fat, 84.9g

DAY 17	
BreakFast	Chocolate and Hazelnut Smoothie - no.6. - pg.23
Snack a.m	Peanut Butter Chip Cookies - no.27. - pg.31
Lunch	Sweet Chickpea and Mushroom Stew - no.63. - pg.46
Snack p.m	Grilled Zucchini and Spinach Pizza - no.23. - pg.30
Dinner	Tempeh "Chicken" Salad - no.143. - pg.83
Dessert	Mixed Berry Mousse - no.0 - pg.106

Tot. Nut.	Kcal, 1938	Protein, 93.2g
		Carbs, 172g
		Fat, 147g

DAY 18	
BreakFast	Mint Chocolate Protein Smoothie - no.14. - pg.26
Snack a.m	Kale Bowls - no.26. - pg.31
Lunch	Garlic Mashed Potatoes & Turnips - no.113. - pg.69
Snack p.m	Chickpea Avocado Pizza - no.20. - pg.28
Dinner	Steamed Artichoke with Lemon Aioli - no.139. - pg.81
Dessert	Peanut Butter Bars - no.0 - pg.106

Tot. Nut.	Kcal, 1771	Protein, 81g
		Carbs, 199.5g
		Fat, 91g

DAY 19	
BreakFast	Sweet Potato Breakfast Hash - no.17. - pg.27
Snack a.m	Watermelon Pizza - no.31. - pg.33
Lunch	Anasazi Bean and Vegetable Stew - no.65. - pg.47
Snack p.m	Peanut Butter Chip Cookies - no.27. - pg.31
Dinner	Simple Baked Okra... - no.121. - pg.73
Dessert	Homemade Protein Bar - no.0 - pg.106

Tot. Nut.	Kcal, 1619	Protein, 73g
		Carbs, 126g
		Fat, 74.3g

DAY 20	
BreakFast	Avocado Toast with White Beans - no.1. - pg.21
Snack a.m	Turmeric Snack Bites - no.30. - pg.32
Lunch	Roasted Sweet Potatoes - no.117. - pg.71
Snack p.m	Garden Salad Wraps - no.22. - pg.29
Dinner	Chickpea and Spinach Salad - no.124. - pg.75
Dessert	Rainbow Fruit Salad - no.0 - pg.106

Tot. Nut.	Kcal, 1910	Protein, 68g
		Carbs, 154g
		Fat, 86g

DAY 21	
BreakFast	Chocolate and Peanut Butter Smo... - no.7. - pg.23
Snack a.m	Curried Tofu "Egg Salad" Pitas - no.21. - pg.29
Lunch	Spicy Cheesy Tofu Balls... - no.119. - pg.72
Snack p.m	Risotto Bites - no.28. - pg.32
Dinner	Grilled Veggie and Hummus Wrap - no.129. - pg.77
Dessert	Shortbread Cookies - no.0 - pg.107

Tot. Nut.	Kcal, 1916	Protein, 62.4g
		Carbs, 135g
		Fat, 117g

7. Week 4 Shopping List

- 6.5 fl. oz. Coconut Oil, Unsalted
- 22 fl. oz. Olive Oil
- 2 fl. oz. Avocado Oil
- 2 fl. oz. Walnut Oil
- 1 fl. oz. Vegetable Oil
- 1 fl. oz. Toasted Sesame Oil
- 32 fl. oz. Almond Milk
- 10 oz. Almond Butter
- 1.5 lb. Almond Flour
- 2.5 oz. Cacao Nibs +4 oz. Raw Cacao Powder
- 4 oz. Coconut Flakes, Unsweetened
- ⅓ Cup Erythritol
- ¼ Cup Nut Butter
- 1 lb. Potatoes
- 16 fl. oz. Vegetable Broth
- 10 Carrots
- 3 Celery Stalks & 2 Ribs
- 2.5 lb. Onions
- 1 lb. Red Onion
- ½ tsp. Onion Powder
- 3 Zucchinis
- 10 oz. Feta Cheese
- 8 oz. Tofu Cheese
- 6 oz. Vegan Parmesan Cheese
- 2 lb. Asparagus Spears
- 2.5 lb. Cauliflower Florets
- 1 Small Head of Broccoli
- 9 oz. Rice Broccoli
- 5 oz. Green Beans
- 1 Chopped Turnip Greens
- 25 Cherry Tomatoes
- 3 Ripe Roma Tomatoes
- 3 Tomatoes + 28 oz. Canned & Crushed Tomatoes
- 25 Grape Tomatoes
- 2½ Cabbages
- 1 oz. Pod
- 3 lb. Extra-Firm Tofu
- 1 Medium Red Pepper
- 4 Medium Avocados
- 4 Ripe Hass Avocados
- 1 Head Garlic
- 1 Tbsp. Ground Turmeric
- 1 Small Packet of Ground Black Pepper & Salt
- 1/4 Teaspoon Cumin
- 8 Corn Tortillas
- 8 (10-Inch) Whole-Grain Flour Tortillas or Lavash Flatbread
- 10 Frozen Bananas + 2 Fresh Bananas
- 8 oz. Kale
- 12 oz. Peanut Butter

- 40 fl. oz. Coconut Milk, Unsweetened
- 4 fl. oz. Unsweetened Soy Milk
- ½ Cup Swerve
- 2 fl. oz Vanilla Extract
- 32 oz. Whole-Wheat Flour
- 4 oz. Flax Seed Powder
- 3 Tbsp. Pure Malt Syrup
- 5 oz. Vegan Butter
- 10 oz. Cashew Cream
- 6 Tbsp. Pure Date Sugar
- 1 Cup Mixed Frozen Berries
- 9 oz. Sugar-Free Chocolate Chips
- Stevia, To Taste
- 15 oz. Pecans
- 16 oz. Vegan Mayonnaise, Homemade or Store-Bought
- 2 Scallions
- 4 ½ Cups Mixed Salad Greens
- 2 oz. White Miso
- 2 oz. Chopped Fresh Dill
- 7 oz. Crumbled Tempeh
- 3 Cans (15 oz.) White Beans
- 1 Large Eggplant
- 6 Lavash Wraps or Large Pita Bread
- 1 Cup Creamy Traditional Hummus
- 2 lb. Large Acorn Squash
- 10 oz. Spinach
- ½ Cup Vegetable Stock
- 4.5 oz. Medjool Dates
- 3 oz. Walnuts
- 1 Tbsp. Cocoa Powder, Unsweetened
- 1 Small Packet Ground Cinnamon
- ½ Cup Panko Breadcrumbs
- 1 tsp. Paprika
- 1 tsp. Chipotle Powder or Ground Cayenne Pepper
- 10 oz. Cold Green Pea Risotto
- 0.6 lb. Almonds
- 6 Lemons
- ⅔ Cup Jarred Roasted Peppers
- 1 tsp. Italian Seasoning
- ¼ tsp. Chili Powder
- 1 oz. Yeast
- 1 Cup Red Pizza Sauce
- 1 (15 oz.) Can of Chickpeas
- 3 oz. Coconut Sugar
- 14 oz. Rolled Oats
- 16 oz. Porridge Oats
- 4 oz. Chia Seeds
- ½ Cup Sun-Butter

- ½ Cup Apple Sauce
- 3 Fresh Mangoes
- 7 Fresh Limes, Juiced
- 2 Fresh Mint Sprigs
- ½ Cup Popcorn Kernels
- 1.5 oz. Honey
- 1 oz. Tamari or Soy Sauce
- ¾ Cup Brown Rice
- 2 oz. Ginger
- 1 Bell Pepper
- 1 Tbsp. Curry Powder
- 4 Cod Filets
- 2.5 oz. Cilantro
- 5 oz. Parsley
- 12 oz. Arugula
- 4 oz. Black Olives
- 2 oz. Green Olives
- 1 lb. Brussels Sprouts
- 2 oz. Soy Sauce
- ¼ Cup Coconut Water
- 1 Tbsp. Sesame Seeds
- 4 Slices Rye Bread, Toasted
- 1 Tbsp. Pumpkin Seeds
- 6 oz. Raspberries
- 8 oz. Tempeh Bacon, Homemade or Store-Bought
- 4 Large Lettuce Leaves
- 3 Cups Shredded Romaine Lettuce
- 8 Small Boston or Other Soft Lettuce Leaves
- ¼ Cup Mango Chutney, Homemade or Store-Bought
- 3 tsp. Dijon Mustard
- 1 Tbsp. Hot or Mild Curry Powder
- ⅛ tsp. Ground Cayenne
- 4 (7-Inch) Whole-Wheat Pita Bread, Halved
- 1 Cup Marinara Sauce
- 1 Jicama Bulb
- 1 tsp. Baking Soda
- 10 fl. oz. Apple Cider Vinegar
- 1 Medium English Cucumber
- ½ Cup Strawberries
- 16 oz. Blueberries
- 1 Watermelon
- 12 oz. Coconut Yogurt
- ½ Cup Pomegranate Seeds
- ½ Cup Cherries
- 1 Bottle Maple Syrup
- 8 oz. Plain Flour
- 1 tsp. Baking Powder
- 10 oz. Tempeh Slices
- ¼ tsp. Nutmeg
- ¼ Cup Nuts Seeds

8. Week 4 Meal Plan

DAY 22	
BreakFast	Kale and Peanut Butter Smoothie - no.11. - pg.25
Snack a.m	Avocado and Tempeh Bacon Wraps - no.19. - pg.28
Lunch	Cauliflower Salad - no.106. - pg.66
Snack p.m	Curried Tofu "Egg Salad" Pitas - no.21. - pg.29
Dinner	Tempeh "Chicken" Salad... - no.143. - pg.83
Dessert	Tropical Cookies - no.0 - pg.107

Tot. Nut.	*Kcal, 1996*	Protein, 92g
		Carbs, 154g
		Fat, 106g

DAY 23	
BreakFast	Overnight Oats - no.15. - pg.26
Snack a.m	Chickpea Avocado Pizza - no.20. - pg.28
Lunch	Coconut Brussels sprouts - no.108. - pg.67
Snack p.m	Grilled Zucchini and Spinach ... - no.23. - pg.30
Dinner	Steamed Artichoke with Lemon Aioli - no.139. - pg.81
Dessert	Peanut Butter Bars... - no.0 - pg.106

Tot. Nut.	*Kcal, 1825.6*	Protein, 72g
		Carbs, 246g
		Fat, 96g

DAY 24	
BreakFast	Super Smoothie - no.18. - pg.27
Snack a.m	Garden Salad Wraps - no.22. - pg.29
Lunch	Cod Stew with Rice & Sweet Potatoes - no.110. - pg.68
Snack p.m	Honey-Almond Popcorn - no.24. - pg.30
Dinner	Vegetable Medley - no.126. - pg.76
Dessert	Mini Berry Tarts - no.0 - pg.105

Tot. Nut.	*Kcal, 2094*	Protein, 80g
		Carbs, 190g
		Fat, 71g

DAY 25	
BreakFast	High Protein Toast - no.9. - pg.24
Snack a.m	Jicama and Guacamole - no.25. - pg.31
Lunch	Curry Mushroom Pie - no.112. - pg.69
Snack p.m	Peanut Butter Chip Cookies - no.27. - pg.31
Dinner	Asparagus with Feta - no.122. - pg.74
Dessert	Crunchy Bars - no.196. - pg.104

Tot. Nut.	*Kcal, 1747*	Protein, 93.5g
		Carbs, 144g
		Fat, 161.5g

DAY 26	
BreakFast	Scrambled Tofu Breakfast Tacos - no.12. - pg.25
Snack a.m	Kale Bowls - no.26. - pg.31
Lunch	Pecan & Blueberry Crumble - no.115. - pg.70
Snack p.m	Risotto Bites - no.28. - pg.32
Dinner	Greek Style Beans - no.128. - pg.77
Dessert	Banana Ice Cream - no.190. - pg.102

Tot. Nut.	*Kcal, 1600*	Protein, 61.8g
		Carbs, 97.9g
		Fat, 89.7g

DAY 27	
BreakFast	Sun-Butter Baked Oatmeal Cups - no.16. - pg.27
Snack a.m	Tamari Toasted Almonds - no.29. - pg.32
Lunch	Dry Belly Soup Recipe with Cabbage - no.67. - pg.48
Snack p.m	Watermelon Pizza - no.31. - pg.33
Dinner	Grilled Veggie and Hummus Wrap... - no.129. - pg.77
Dessert	Avocado Pudding - no.189. - pg.101

Tot. Nut.	*Kcal, 1554*	Protein, 70.7g
		Carbs, 83.2g
		Fat, 34.8g

DAY 28	
BreakFast	Mango Agua Fresca... - no.13. - pg.25
Snack a.m	Turmeric Snack Bites - no.30. - pg.32
Lunch	Smoked Tempeh with Broccoli Fri... - no.118. - pg.71
Snack p.m	White Bean Stuffed Squash - no.32. - pg.33
Dinner	Spinach & Dill Pasta Salad - no.138. - pg.81
Dessert	Apple Almond Slush - no.188. - pg.101

Tot. Nut.	*Kcal, 1905*	Protein, 69g
		Carbs, 137.1g
		Fat, 112g

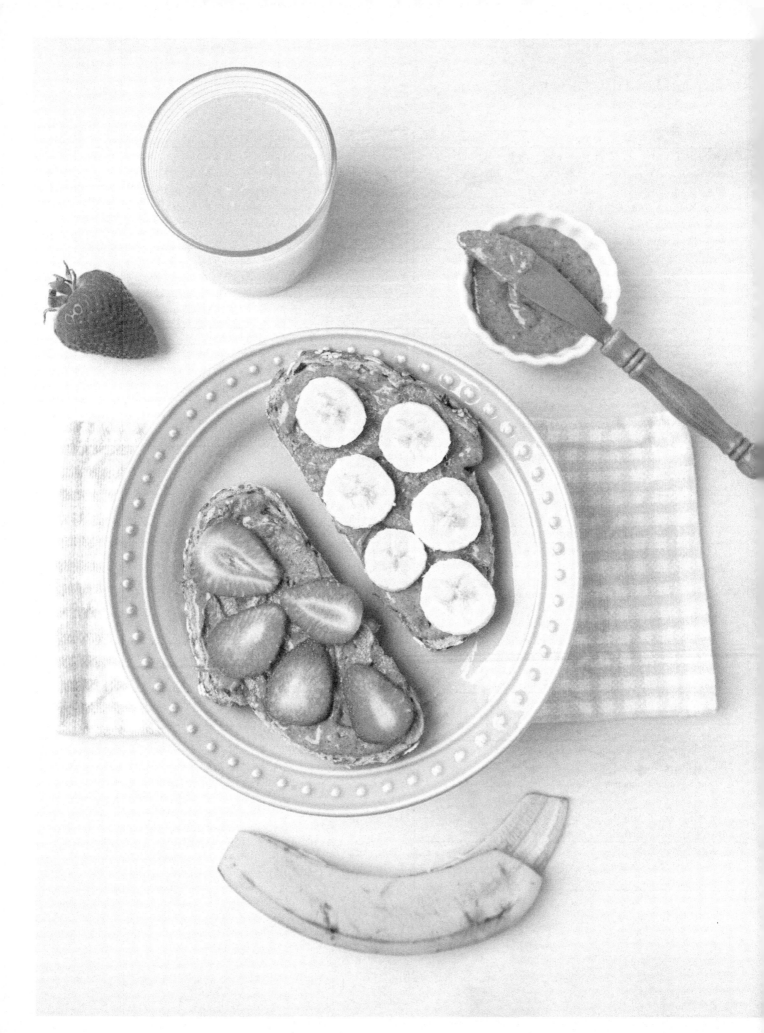

Chapter 5: Breakfast and Smoothies

1. Avocado Toast with White Beans

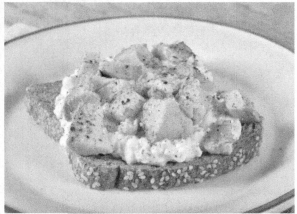

Preparation Time: 5 minutes, **Cooking Time:** 6 minutes, **Difficulty Level:** Easy, **Servings:** 4

Ingredients:
- ½ cup canned white beans, drained and rinsed
- 2 tsp. Tahini paste
- 2 tsp. lemon juice
- ½ tsp. salt
- ½ avocado, peeled and pit removed
- 4 slices whole-grain bread, toasted
- ½ cup grape tomatoes, cut in half

Directions:
1. Grab a small bowl and add the beans, Tahini, ½ the lemon juice, and ½ the salt. Mash with a fork.
2. In another bowl, add the avocado, the remaining lemon juice and the rest of the salt. Mash together.
3. Place your toast onto a flat surface and add the mashed beans, spreading well.
4. Top with the avocado and the sliced tomatoes, then serve and enjoy.

Nutrition: Calories: 140 kcal, Fat: 5.0 g, Carbs: 13.0 g, Protein: 5.0 g

2. Banana and Chai Chia Smoothie

Preparation Time: 5 minutes, **Cooking Time:** 0 minutes, **Difficulty Level:** Easy, **Servings:** 4

Ingredients:
- 1 banana
- 1 cup alfalfa sprouts
- 1 Tbsp. chia seeds
- ½ cup unsweetened coconut milk
- 1 to 2 soft Medjool dates, pitted
- ¼ tsp. ground cinnamon
- 1 Tbsp. grated fresh ginger
- 1 cup water
- A pinch ground cardamom

Directions:
1. First, place all of the ingredients for the smoothie into a blender, then process until the mixture is smooth and creamy. Add water or coconut milk if necessary.
2. Serve immediately.

Nutrition: Calories: 477 kcal, Fat: 41.0 g, Carbs: 31.0 g, Fiber: 14.0 g, Protein: 17.5 g

3. Berries and Banana Smoothie Bowl

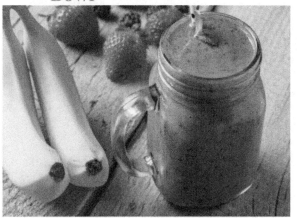

Preparation Time: 5 minutes, **Cooking Time:** 0 minutes, **Difficulty Level:** Easy, **Servings:** 4

Ingredients:
For the Smoothie:
- 4 cups frozen mixed berries
- 4 small frozen bananas, sliced
- 4 scoops of vanilla protein powder
- 12 Tbsp. Almond milk, unsweetened

For the Toppings:
- 4 Tbsp. Chia seeds
- 4 Tbsp. shredded coconut, unsweetened
- 4 Tbsp. Hemp seeds
- ½ cup Granola
- Fresh strawberries, sliced, as needed

Directions:
1. Add mixed berries into a food processor and banana and then pulse at low speed for 1 to 2 minutes until broken.

2. Add remaining ingredients for the smoothie and then pulse again for 1 minute at low speed until creamy, scraping the sides of the container frequently.
3. Distribute the smoothie among four bowls, then top with chia seeds, coconut, hemp seeds, granola, and strawberries. Serve.

Nutrition: Calories: 214 kcal, Fat: 2.5 g, Saturated Fat: 1.6 g, Carbohydrates: 47.5 g, Fiber: 8.8 g, Sugars: 26 g, Protein: 2.8 g

4. Broccoli and Quinoa Breakfast Patties

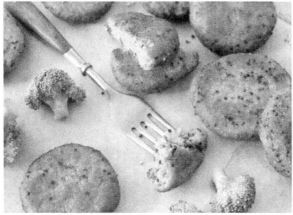

Preparation Time: 5 minutes, **Cooking Time:** 6 minutes, **Difficulty Level:** Easy, **Serving:** 4

Ingredients:
- 1 cup cooked quinoa, cooked
- 1/2 cup shredded broccoli florets
- 1/2 cup shredded carrots
- 2 cloves of garlic, minced
- 2 teaspoon parsley
- 1 1/2 teaspoon onion powder
- 1 1/2 teaspoon garlic powder
- 1/3 teaspoon salt
- 1/4 teaspoon black pepper
- 1/2 cup bread crumbs, gluten-free
- 2 tablespoon coconut oil
- 2 flax eggs

Directions:
1. Prepare patties and for this, place all the ingredients in a large bowl, except for oil, and stir until well mixed and then shape the mixture into patties.
2. Take a skillet pan, place it over medium heat, add oil and when hot, add prepared patties in it and cook for 3 MIN. per side until golden brown and crispy.
3. Serve patties with vegan sour creams.

Nutrition: Calories: 229.6 kcal, Fat: 11.1 g, Carbs: 27.7g, Protein: 9.3g, Fiber: 6.6 g

5. Blueberry Oatmeal Smoothie

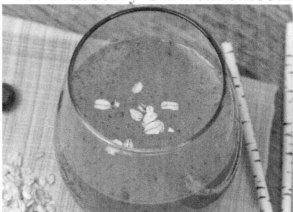

Preparation Time: 5 minutes, **Cooking Time:** 0 minutes, **Difficulty Level:** Easy, **Servings:** 4

Ingredients:
- 2 cups frozen blueberries
- 1 cup old-fashioned oats
- 2 tsp. cinnamon
- 2 Tbsp. maple syrup
- 1 cup spinach
- 2 cup almond milk, unsweetened
- 8 ice cubes

Directions:
1. Add all the ingredients in the order into a food processor or blender and then pulse for 1 to 2 minutes until blended, scraping the sides of the container frequently.
2. Distribute the smoothie among glasses and then serve.

Nutrition: Calories: 194 kcal, Fat: 5.0 g, Saturated Fat: 3.0 g, Carbohydrates: 34.0 g, Fiber: 5.0 g, Sugars: 15.0 g, Protein: 5.0 g

6. Chocolate and Hazelnut Smoothie

Preparation Time: 5 minutes, **Cooking Time:** 0 minutes, **Difficulty Level:** Easy, **Servings:** 4

Ingredients:
- 1 frozen banana
- 1 cup hazelnuts, unsalted, roasted
- 8 tsp. maple syrup
- 4 Tbsp. cocoa powder, unsweetened
- ½ tsp. hazelnut extract, unsweetened
- 2 cups almond milk, unsweetened
- 1 cup of ice cubes

Directions:
1. Add all the ingredients, in the order, into a food processor or blender and then pulse for 1 to 2 minutes until blended, scraping the sides of the container frequently.
2. Distribute the smoothie among glasses and then serve.

Nutrition: Calories: 198 kcal, Fat: 12.0 g, Saturated Fat: 1.0 g, Carbohydrates: 21.0 g, Fiber: 5.0 g, Sugars: 12.0 g, Protein: 5.0 g

7. Chocolate and Peanut Butter Smoothie

Preparation Time: 5 minutes, **Cooking Time:** 0 minutes, **Difficulty Level:** Easy, **Servings:** 4

Ingredients:
- 1 Tbsp. unsweetened cocoa powder
- 1 Tbsp. peanut butter
- 1 banana
- 1 tsp. maca powder
- ½ cup unsweetened soy milk
- ¼ cup rolled oats
- 1 Tbsp. flaxseeds
- 1 Tbsp. maple syrup
- 1 cup water

Directions:
1. First, place all of the ingredients for the smoothie into a blender, then process until the mixture is smooth and creamy. Add water or soy milk if necessary.
2. Serve immediately.

Nutrition: Calories: 474 kcal, Fat: 16.0 g, Carbs: 27.0 g, Fiber: 18.0 g, Protein: 13.0 g

8. Chocolate Chip Banana Pancake

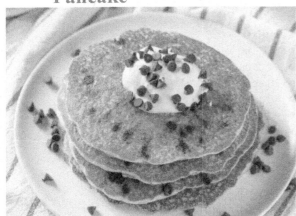

Preparation Time: 15 minutes, **Cooking Time:** 5 minutes, **Difficulty Level:** Moderate, **Servings:** 4

Ingredients:
- 1 large ripe banana, mashed
- 2 Tbsp. coconut sugar
- 3 Tbsp. coconut oil, melted
- 1 cup of coconut milk
- 1 ½ cups whole wheat flour
- 1 tsp. baking soda
- ½ cup vegan chocolate chips
- Olive oil, for frying

Directions:
1. Grab a large bowl and add the banana, sugar, oil, and milk. Stir well.
2. Add the flour and baking soda and stir again until combined.
3. Add the chocolate chips and fold through, then pop to one side.
4. Put a skillet over medium heat and add a drop of oil.
5. Pour ¼ of the batter into the pan and move the pan to cover.
6. Cook for 3 minutes, then flip and cook on the other side.
7. Repeat with the remaining pancakes, then serve and enjoy.

Nutrition: Calories: 105 kcal, Fat: 13.0 g, Carbs: 23.0 g, Protein: 5.0 g

9. High Protein Toast

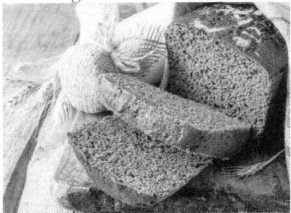

Preparation Time: 15 minutes, **Cooking Time:** 15 minutes, **Difficulty Level:** Moderate, **Servings:** 4

Ingredients:
- 1 white bean, drained and rinsed
- ½ cup cashew cream
- 1 ½ Tbsp. miso paste
- 1 tsp. toasted sesame oil
- 1 Tbsp. sesame seeds

- 1 spring onion, finely sliced
- 1 lemon, half for the juice, and half wedged to serve
- 4 slices rye bread, toasted

Directions:
1. In a bowl, add sesame oil, white beans, miso, cashew cream, and lemon juice and mash using a potato masher
2. Make a spread
3. Spread it on a toast and top with spring onions and sesame seeds
4. Serve with lemon wedges

Nutrition: Carbs: 44.05 g, Protein: 14. 05 g, Fats: 9. 25 g, Calories: 332 kcal

10. Hummus Carrot Sandwich

Preparation Time: 15 minutes, **Cooking Time:** 25 minutes, **Difficulty Level:** Moderate, **Servings:** 4

Ingredients:
- 1 cup chickpeas, drained and rinsed
- 1 small tomato, sliced
- 1 cucumber, sliced
- 1 avocado, sliced
- 1 tsp. cumin
- 1 cup carrot, diced
- 1 tsp. maple syrup
- 3 Tbsp. Tahini
- 1 clove garlic
- 2 Tbsp. Lemon
- 2 Tbsp. extra-virgin oil
- Salt, as per your need
- 4 slices of bread

Directions:
1. Add carrot to the boiling hot water and boil for 15 minutes
2. Blend boiled carrots, maple syrup, cumin, chickpeas, tahini, olive oil, salt, and garlic in a blender
3. Add in lemon juice and mix
4. Add to a serving bowl. It can be refrigerated for up to 5 days
5. Take a slice of bread. Spread some hummus on it, then place 2-3 slices of cucumber, avocado and tomato. Spread hummus on another slice of bread, place it on top of the other slice, and the sandwich is ready to serve.

Nutrition: Carbs: 53.15 g, Protein: 14.1 g, Fats: 27.5 g, Calories: 490 kcal

11. Kale and Peanut Butter Smoothie

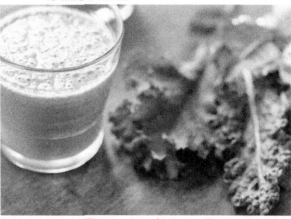

Preparation Time: 5 minutes, **Cooking Time:** 0 minutes, **Difficulty Level:** Easy, **Servings:** 4

Ingredients:
- 4 frozen bananas, sliced
- 2 cups kale
- ½ cup peanut butter
- 2 ⅔ cups coconut milk, unsweetened

Directions:
1. Add all the ingredients in the order into a food processor or blender and then pulse for 1 to 2 minutes until blended, scraping the sides of the container frequently.
2. Distribute the smoothie among glasses and then serve.

Nutrition: Calories: 390 kcal, Fat: 19.0 g, Saturated Fat: 2.5 g, Carbohydrates: 42.0 g, Fiber: 7.0 g, Sugars: 22.0 g, Protein: 15.0 g

12. Scrambled Tofu Breakfast Tacos

Preparation Time: 5 minutes, **Cooking Time:** 10 minutes, **Difficulty Level:** Easy, **Serving:** 4

Ingredients:
- 12 oz. tofu, pressed, drained
- 1/2 cup grape tomatoes, quartered
- 1 medium red pepper, diced
- 1 medium avocado, sliced
- 1 garlic clove, minced
- 1/4 teaspoon ground turmeric
- 1/4 teaspoon ground black pepper
- 1/4 teaspoon salt
- 1/4 teaspoon cumin
- 1 teaspoon olive oil
- 8 corn tortillas

Directions:
1. Take a skillet pan, place it over medium heat, add oil and when hot, add pepper and garlic. Cook for 2 minutes.
2. Then add tofu, crumble it, sprinkle it with black pepper, salt, and all the spices, stir and cook for 5 minutes.
3. When done, distribute tofu between tortilla, top with tomato and avocado, and serve.

Nutrition: Calories: 316 kcal, Fat: 14.4 g, Carbs: 37.6 g, Protein: 22.5 g, Fiber: 8 g

13.   Mango Agua Fresca

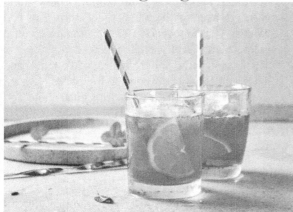

Preparation Time: 5 minutes, **Cooking Time:** 0 minutes, **Difficulty Level:** Easy, **Servings:** 4

Ingredients:
- 2 fresh mangoes, diced
- 1½ cups water
- 1 tsp. fresh lime juice
- Maple syrup, to taste
- 2 cups ice
- 2 slices fresh lime for garnish
- 2 fresh mint sprigs for garnish

Directions:
1. Put the mangoes, lime juice, maple syrup, and water in a blender. Process until creamy and smooth.
2. Divide the beverage into two glasses, then garnish each glass with ice, lime slice, and mint sprig before serving.

Nutrition: Calories: 230 kcal, Fat: 1.3 g, Carbs: 57.7 g, Fiber: 5.4 g, Protein: 16 g

14.   Mint Chocolate Protein Smoothie

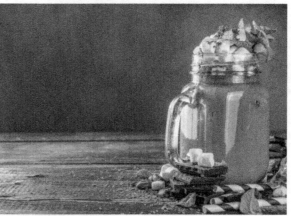

Preparation Time: 5 minutes, **Cooking Time:** 0 minutes, **Difficulty Level:** Easy, **Servings:** 4

Ingredients:
- 4 Tbsp. ground flaxseed
- 4 cups fresh spinach
- 4 frozen bananas, sliced
- 4 scoops of chocolate protein powder
- 4 Tbsp. chopped dark chocolate, vegan
- ½ cup melted dark chocolate
- 1 tsp. peppermint extract, unsweetened
- 4 Tbsp. Honey
- 3 cups almond milk, unsweetened
- 1 cup ice cubed

Directions:
1. Add all the ingredients in the order into a food processor or blender and then pulse for 1 to 2 minutes until blended, scraping the sides of the container frequently.
2. Distribute the smoothie among glasses and then serve.

Nutrition: Calories: 480.5 kcal, Fat: 20.3 g, Saturated Fat: 8.4 g, Carbohydrates: 45.6 g, Fiber: 9.7 g, Sugars: 22.5 g, Protein: 31.2 g

15.   Overnight Oats

Preparation Time: 10 minutes, **Cooking Time:** 0 minutes, **Difficulty Level:** Easy, **Servings:** 4

Ingredients:
- A pinch cinnamon
- 2 ½ cups almond milk
- 3 ½ cups porridge oats
- 1 Tbsp. maple syrup
- 1 Tbsp. pumpkin seeds
- 1 Tbsp. chia seeds

Directions:

1. First, add all the ingredients for the oats to the bowl and combine well
2. Then cover the bowl and place in the fridge overnight
3. Pour more milk in the morning. Serve with your favorite toppings

Nutrition: Carbs: 32.3 g, Protein: 10.2 g, Fats: 12.7 g, Calories: 298 kcal

16.   Sun-Butter Baked Oatmeal Cups

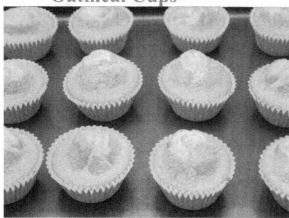

Preparation Time: 10 minutes, **Cooking Time:** 35 minutes, **Difficulty Level:** Easy, **Servings:** 4

Ingredients:
- ¼ cup coconut sugar
- 1 ½ rolled oats
- 2 Tbsp. chia seeds
- ¼ tsp. salt
- 1 tsp. cinnamon
- ½ cup non-dairy milk
- ½ cup Sun-Butter
- ½ cup apple sauce

Directions:
1. Preheat oven to 350 °F.
2. Mix all ingredients and blend well.
3. Add in muffins and insert extra toppings, then bake for 25 minutes or until they turn golden brown.

Nutrition: Calories: 129 kcal, Fat: 1.1 g, Carbohydrates: 1.5 g, Protein: 4.9 g

17.   Sweet Potato Breakfast Hash

Preparation Time: 5 minutes, **Cooking Time:** 28 minutes, **Difficulty Level:** Easy, **Serves:** 4

Ingredients:
- 4 cups cubed sweet potatoes, peeled
- 1/2 teaspoon sea salt
- 1/2 teaspoon turmeric
- 1/2 teaspoon cumin
- 1 teaspoon smoked paprika
- 2 cups diced white onion
- 2 garlic cloves, peeled, minced
- 1/4 cup chopped cilantro
- 1 tablespoon coconut oil
- ½ cup vegan guacamole, for serving
- 1 ½ cup Pico de Gallo

Directions:
1. Take a skillet pan, place it over medium heat, add oil and when it melts, add onion, potatoes, and garlic, season with salt, paprika, turmeric, and cumin, stir and cook for 25 minutes. until potatoes are slightly caramelized.
2. Then, remove the pan from heat, add cilantro and distribute evenly between serving plates.
3. Top the sweet potato hash with guacamole and Pica de Gallo, and then serve.

Nutrition: Calories: 211.3 kcal, Fat: 8 g, Carbs: 22.2 g, Protein: 12.5 g, Fiber: 3.5 g

18.   Super Smoothie

Preparation Time: 5 minutes, **Cooking Time:** 0 minutes, **Difficulty Level:** Easy, **Servings:** 4

Ingredients:
- 1 banana, peeled
- 1 cup chopped mango
- 1 cup raspberries
- ¼ cup rolled oats
- 1 carrot, peeled
- 1 cup chopped fresh kale
- 2 Tbsp. chopped fresh parsley
- 1 Tbsp. flaxseeds
- 1 Tbsp. grated fresh ginger
- ½ cup unsweetened soy milk
- 1 cup water

Directions:
1. First, put all the ingredients of the smoothie in a food processor, then blitz until glossy and smooth.
2. You may serve immediately or chill in the refrigerator for an hour before serving.

Nutrition: Calories: 126 kcal, Fat: 2.2 g, Carbs: 25.0 g, Fiber: 5.7 g, Protein: 4 g

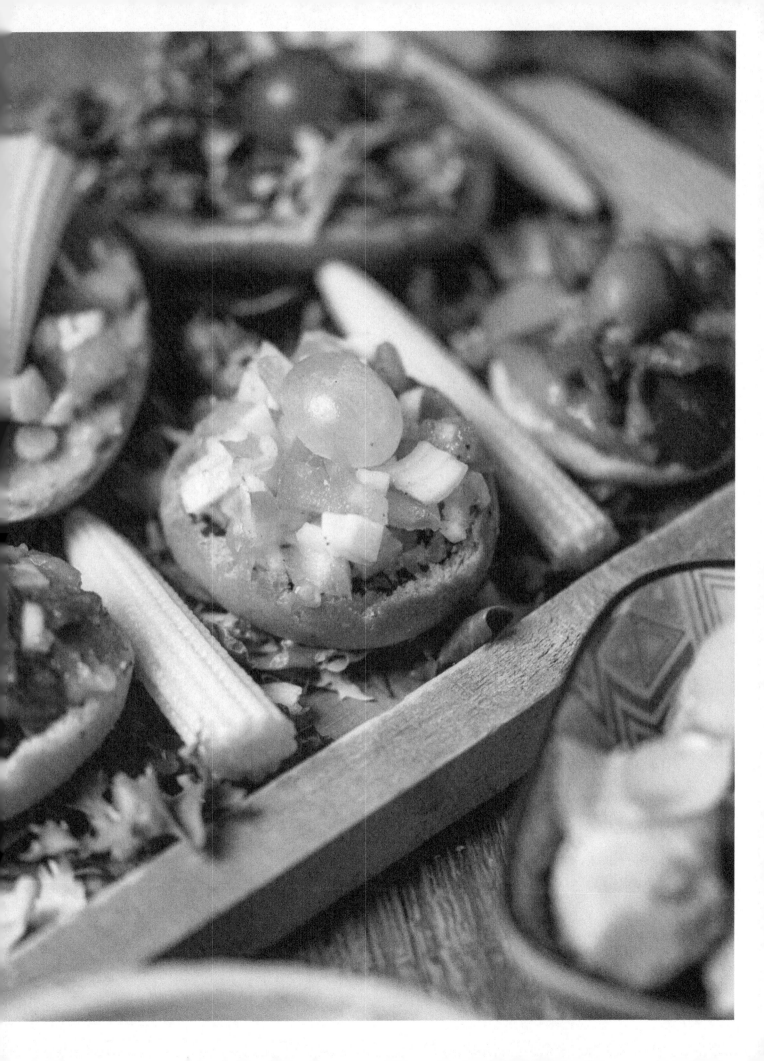

Chapter 6: Snack and Appetizers

19. Avocado and Tempeh Bacon Wraps

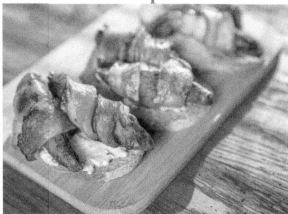

Preparation Time: 10 minutes, **Cooking Time:** 8, minutes, **Difficulty Level:** Moderate, **Servings:** 4

Ingredients:
- 2 Tbsp. olive oil
- 8 oz. tempeh bacon, homemade or store-bought
- 4 (10-inch) soft flour tortillas or lavash flatbread
- 1/4 cup vegan mayonnaise, homemade or store-bought
- 4 large lettuce leaves
- 2 ripe Hass avocados, pitted, peeled, and cut into 1/4-inch slices
- 1 large ripe tomato, cut into 1/4-inch slices

Directions:
1. Heat the oil in a large skillet over medium heat. Add the tempeh bacon and cook until browned on both sides, about 8 minutes. Remove from the heat and set aside.
2. Place 1 tortilla on a work surface. Spread with some of the mayonnaise and one-fourth of the lettuce and tomatoes.
3. Pit, peel, and thinly slice the avocado and place the slices on top of the tomato. Add the reserved tempeh bacon and roll up tightly. Repeat with remaining ingredients and serve.

Nutrition: Calories: 379 kcal, Fat: 5.0 g, Carbs: 6.0 g Fiber: 2.0 g, Protein: 18.05 g

20. Chickpea Avocado Pizza

Preparation Time: 15-30 minutes, **Cooking Time:** 40 minutes, **Difficulty Level:** Hard, **Servings:** 4

Ingredients:
For the Pizza Crust:
- 3 ½ cups whole-wheat flour
- 1 tsp. yeast
- 1 tsp. salt
- A pinch sugar
- 3 Tbsp. olive oil
- 1 cup warm water

For the Topping:
- 1 cup red pizza sauce
- 1 cup baby spinach
- 1 (15 oz.) can of chickpeas, rinsed and drained
- Salt and black pepper, to taste
- 1 medium avocado, pitted, peeled, and chopped
- ¼ cup grated plant-based Parmesan cheese

Directions:
1. Preheat the oven to 350 °F and lightly grease a pizza pan with cooking spray.
2. Mix the flour, nutritional yeast, salt, sugar, olive oil, and warm water until smooth dough forms in a medium bowl. Allow rising for an hour or until the dough doubles in size.
3. Spread the dough onto the pizza pan, then apply the pizza sauce on top.
4. Top with spinach, chickpeas, avocado, and plant Parmesan cheese.
5. For 20 minutes or until the cheese melts, bake the pizza.
6. Remove from the oven, cool for 5 minutes, slice, and serve.

Nutrition: Calories: 678 kcal, Fats: 22.7 g, Carbs: 104.1 g, Protein: 23.5 g

21. Curried Tofu "Egg Salad" Pitas

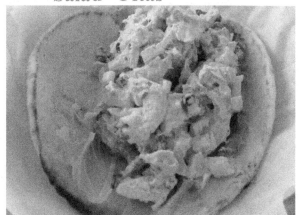

Preparation Time: 15 minutes, **Cooking Time:** 0, minutes, **Difficulty Level:** Moderate, **Servings:** 4

Ingredients:
- 1- oz. extra-firm tofu drained and patted dry
- ½ cup vegan mayonnaise, homemade or store-bought
- ¼ cup chopped mango chutney, homemade or store-bought
- 2 tsp. Dijon mustard
- 1 Tbsp. hot or mild curry powder
- 1 tsp. salt
- ⅛ tsp. ground cayenne
- ¾ cup shredded carrots
- 2 celery ribs, minced
- ¼ cup minced red onion
- 8 small Boston or other soft lettuce leaves
- 4 (7-inch) whole-wheat pita bread, halved

Directions:
1. Crumble the tofu and place the crumbled pieces in a large bowl. Add the mayonnaise, chutney, mustard, curry powder, salt, and cayenne, and stir well until thoroughly mixed.
2. Add the carrots, celery, and onion and stir to combine. Refrigerate for 30 minutes to allow the flavors to blend.
3. Tuck a lettuce leaf inside each pita pocket, spoon some tofu mixture on the lettuce, and serve.

Nutrition: Calories: 435 kcal, Fats: 25 g, Carbs: 37.44 g, Protein: 16 g

22. Garden Salad Wraps

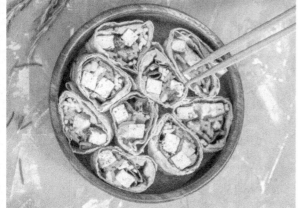

Preparation Time: 15 minutes, **Cooking Time:** 10 minutes, **Difficulty Level:** Moderate, **Servings:** 4

Ingredients:
- 6 Tbsp. olive oil
- 1 lb. extra-firm tofu, drained, patted dry, and cut into 1⁄2-inch strips
- 1 Tbsp. soy sauce

- ¼ cup apple cider vinegar
- 1 tsp. yellow or spicy brown mustard
- ½ tsp. salt
- ¼ tsp. freshly ground black pepper
- 3 cups shredded romaine lettuce
- 3 ripe Roma tomatoes, finely chopped
- 1 large carrot, shredded
- 1 medium English cucumber, peeled and chopped
- ⅓ cup minced red onion
- ¼ cup sliced pitted green olives
-
- 4 (10-inch) whole-grain flour tortillas or lavash flatbread

Directions:
1. In a large skillet, heat only 2 tablespoons of the oil over medium heat. Add the tofu and cook until golden brown, about 10 minutes. Sprinkle soy sauce and set aside to cool.
2. In a small bowl, combine the vinegar, mustard, salt, and pepper with the remaining 4 tablespoons of oil, stirring to blend well. Set aside.
3. Combine the lettuce, tomatoes, carrot, cucumber, onion, and olives in a large bowl. Evenly pour the dressing over this and toss to coat.
4. Place 1 tortilla on a work surface and spread with about one-quarter of the salad to assemble wraps. Place a few strips of tofu on the tortilla and roll up tightly. Slice in half.

Nutrition: Calories: 484 kcal, Fats: 33g, Carbs: 30.22g, Protein: 17.45 g

23. Grilled Zucchini and Spinach Pizza

Preparation Time: 15-30 minutes, **Cooking Time:** 30 minutes, **Difficulty Level:** Hard, **Servings:** 4

Ingredients:
For the Pizza Crust:
- 3 ½ cups whole-wheat flour
- 1 tsp. yeast
- 1 tsp. salt
- 1 pinch sugar
- 3 Tbsp. olive oil
- 1 cup warm water

For the Topping:
- 1 cup marinara sauce
- 2 large zucchinis, sliced
- ½ cup chopped spinach
- ¼ cup pitted and sliced black olives
- ½ cup grated plant parmesan cheese

Directions:
1. Preheat the oven to 350 °F and lightly grease a pizza pan with cooking spray.
2. Mix the flour, nutritional yeast, salt, sugar, olive oil, and warm water until smooth dough forms in a medium bowl. Allow rising for an hour or until the dough doubles in size. On the pizza pan, spread the dough and apply the pizza sauce on top.
3. Over medium heat, heat a grill pan. Season the zucchinis with salt, black pepper, and cook in the pan until slightly charred on both sides.
4. Set the cucumbers on the pizza crust and top with spinach, olives, and plant parmesan cheese. Bake for up to 20 minutes or at least until the cheese melts. Remove from the oven, cool for 5 minutes, slice, and serve.

Nutrition: Calories: 519 kcal, Fats: 13.4 g, Carbs: 87.5 g, Protein: 19.6 g

24.   Honey-Almond Popcorn
Preparation Time: 5 minutes, **Cooking Time:** 10 minutes, **Difficulty Level:** Moderate, **Servings:** 4

Ingredients:
- ½ cup popcorn kernels
- 2 Tbsp. honey
- ½ tsp. sea salt
- 2 Tbsp. coconut sugar
- 1 cup roasted almonds
- ¼ cup walnut oil

Directions:
1. Take a pot, place it over medium-low heat, add oil and when it melts, add four kernels and wait until they sizzle.
2. Then add the remaining kernel, toss until coated, sprinkle with sugar, drizzle with honey, shut the pot with the lid, and shake the kernels until popped completely, adding almonds halfway.
3. Once all the kernels have popped, season them with salt and serve straight away.

Nutrition: Calories: 496 kcal, Fat: 36 g, Carbs: 19.0 g, Protein: 18 g, Fiber: 6.89 g

25.   Jicama and Guacamole
Preparation Time: 15 minutes, **Cooking Time:** 0 minutes, **Difficulty Level:** Easy, **Servings:** 4

Ingredients:
- 1 lime (juiced), or 1 Tbsp. prepared lime juice
- 2 Hass avocados, peeled, pits removed, and cut into cubes
- ½ tsp. sea salt
- ½ red onion, minced
- 1 garlic clove, minced
- ¼ cup chopped cilantro (optional)
- 1 jicama bulb, peeled and cut into matchsticks

Directions:
1. In a medium bowl, squeeze the lime juice over the top of the avocado and sprinkle with salt.
2. Lightly mash the avocado with a fork. Stir in the onion, garlic, and cilantro, if using.
3. Serve with slices of jicama to dip in guacamole.
4. Place plastic wrap over the bowl of guacamole and refrigerate to store. The guacamole will keep for about 2 days.

Nutrition: Calories: 350 kcal, Fat: 28.0 g, Fiber: 1.0 g, Carbs: 8.0 g, Protein: 22.0 g

26.   Kale Bowls

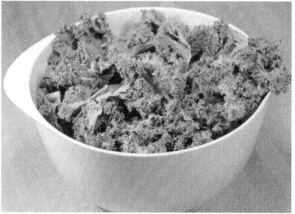

Preparation Time: 10 minutes, **Cooking Time:** 10 minutes, **Difficulty Level:** Easy, **Servings:** 4

Ingredients:
- 2 Tbsp. almonds, chopped
- 2 Tbsp. walnuts, chopped
- 2 bunches kale, trimmed and roughly chopped
- 1 cup cherry tomatoes, halved
- Salt and black pepper, to taste
- 2 Tbsp. avocado oil
- 1 lemon, juiced
- ⅔ cup jarred roasted peppers
- 1 tsp. Italian seasoning
- ¼ tsp. chili powder

Directions:
1. Over medium heat, heat a pan with the oil, then add kale and cook for 5 minutes.
2. Then, add the rest of the ingredients. Toss and cook for 5 minutes more, then divide into bowls and serve as an appetizer.

Nutrition: Calories: 143 kcal, Fat: 5.9 g, Fiber: 4.2 g, Carbs: 9.0 g, Protein: 7.0 g

27.   Peanut Butter Chip Cookies

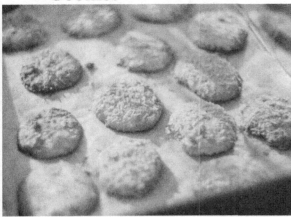

Preparation Time: 10 minutes, **Cooking Time:** 15 minutes, **Difficulty Level:** Moderate, **Servings:** 42

Ingredients:
- 1 Tbsp. ground flaxseed
- 3 Tbsp. hot water
- 1 cup rolled oats
- 1 tsp. baking soda
- 1 tsp. ground cinnamon
- ¼ tsp. salt
- 1 ripe banana, mashed
- ¼ cup maple syrup
- ½ cup all-natural smooth peanut butter
- 1 Tbsp. vanilla extract
- ½ cup dairy-free chocolate chips

Directions:
1. Preheat the oven to 350 °F.
2. Make a flaxseed egg by combining the ground flaxseed and hot water in a small bowl. Stir it thoroughly and wait for it to sit for 5 minutes until thickened.
3. In a medium bowl, combine the oats, baking soda, cinnamon, and salt. Set this aside.
4. Mash the banana and add the maple syrup, peanut butter, flaxseed egg, and vanilla extract in a large bowl. Stir to combine.
5. Add the dry mixture into the wet mixture and stir until just incorporated (do not overmix). Gently fold in the chocolate chips.
6. Drop the cookie dough balls onto the baking sheet using a large spoon or 2-inch ice cream scoop. Flatten them slightly. Bake the peanut butter chip cookies for 12 to 15 minutes or until the bottoms and edges are slightly browned. Serve or store in an airtight container.

Nutrition: Calories: 350 kcal, Fat: 28.0 g, Fiber: 1.0 g, Carbs: 8.0 g, Protein: 22.0 g

28.   Risotto Bites

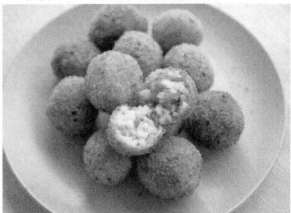

Preparation Time: 15 minutes, **Cooking Time:** 25 minutes, **Difficulty Level:** Moderate, **Servings:** 42

Ingredients:
- ½ cup panko breadcrumbs
- 1 tsp. paprika
- 1 tsp. chipotle powder or ground cayenne pepper
- 1½ cups cold Green Pea Risotto
- Nonstick cooking spray

Directions:
1. Preheat the oven to 425 °F.
2. Line a baking sheet with parchment paper.
3. On a large plate, combine the panko, paprika, and chipotle powder. Set aside.
4. Roll 2 tablespoons of the risotto into a ball.
5. Gently roll in the breadcrumbs and place on the prepared baking sheet. Repeat to make a total of 12 balls.
6. Spritz the tops of the risotto bites with nonstick cooking spray and bake for 15 to 20 minutes until they begin to brown. Before storing in a large airtight container in a single layer (add a piece of parchment paper for a second layer) or in a plastic freezer bag, cool completely.

Nutrition: Calories: 100 kcal, Fat: 2.0 g, Protein: 6.0 g, Carbohydrates: 17.0 g, Fiber: 5.0 g, Sugar: 2.0 g, Sodium: 165 mg

29.   Tamari Toasted Almonds

Preparation Time: 2 minutes, **Cooking Time:** 10 minutes, **Difficulty Level:** Moderate, **Servings:** 4

Ingredients:
- ½ cup raw almonds or sunflower seeds
- 2 Tbsp. tamari or soy sauce
- 1 tsp. toasted sesame oil

Directions:

1. Heat a dry skillet to medium-high heat, then add the almonds, stirring very frequently to keep them from burning. Once the almonds are toasted, 7 to 8 minutes for almonds, or 3 to 4 minutes for sunflower seeds, pour the tamari and sesame oil into the hot skillet and stir to coat.
2. You can turn off the heat, and as the almonds cool, the tamari mixture will stick to and dry on the nuts.

Nutrition (Per Serving): Calories: 140 kcal, Fat: 8.0 g, Carbs: 3.0 g, Fiber: 2.0 g, Protein: 4.0 g

30.   Turmeric Snack Bites

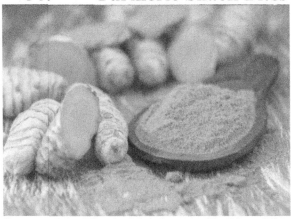

Preparation Time: 35 minutes, **Cooking Time:** 0 minutes, **Difficulty Level:** Easy, **Servings:** 4

Ingredients:
- 1 cup Medjool dates, pitted and chopped
- ½ cup walnuts
- 1 tsp. ground turmeric
- 1 Tbsp. cocoa powder, unsweetened
- ½ tsp. ground cinnamon
- ½ cup shredded coconut, unsweetened

Directions:

1. Place all the ingredients of the turmeric snack bites in a food processor and pulse for 2 minutes until a smooth mixture comes together.
2. Tip the mixture in a bowl and then shape it into ten small balls, 1 tablespoon of the mixture per ball and then refrigerate for 30 minutes.
3. Serve straight away.

Nutrition: Calories: 341 kcal, Fat: 2.0 g, Carbs: 13.0 g, Protein: 6 g, Fiber: 0 g

31.   Watermelon Pizza

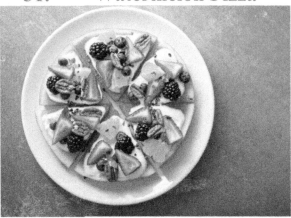

Preparation Time: 10 minutes, **Cooking Time:** 0 minutes, **Difficulty Level:** Easy, **Servings:** 4

Ingredients:
- ½ cup strawberries halved
- ½ cup blueberries
- 1 watermelon
- ½ cup raspberries
- 1 cup coconut yogurt
- ½ cup pomegranate seeds
- ½ cup cherries
- Maple syrup, as needed

Directions:

1. Cut watermelon into 3-inch thick slices, spread yogurt on one side, leaving some space in the edges, and then top evenly with fruits and drizzle with maple syrup.
2. Cut the watermelon into wedges and then serve.

Nutrition: Calories: 386 kcal, Fat: 4.0 g, Carbs: 21.0 g, Protein: 17 g, Fiber: 2.0 g

32.   White Bean Stuffed Squash

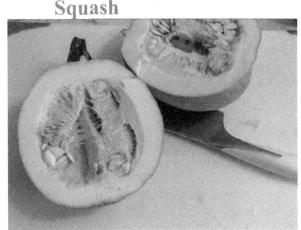

Preparation Time: 15 minutes, **Cooking Time:** 60 minutes, **Difficulty Level:** Hard, **Servings:** 4

Ingredients:

- 2 lb. large acorn squash
- 3 garlic cloves, minced
- 2 Tbsp. olive oil
- 1 (15 oz.) can white beans, drained and rinsed
- 1 cup chopped spinach leaves
- Salt and black pepper, to taste
- ½ cup vegetable stock
- ½ tsp. cumin powder
- ½ tsp. chili powder

Directions:

1. Preheat the oven to 350 °F.
2. Cut the large acorn squash in half and scoop out the seeds.
3. Season with salt and pepper and place face down on a sheet pan. Bake for 45 minutes.
4. While the acorn squash cooks, heat the olive oil in a medium pot over medium heat.
5. Sauté the garlic until fragrant, around 30 seconds, and mix in the beans. Cook for 1 minute.
6. Stir in the spinach, allow wilting for 2 minutes, and season with salt, black pepper, cumin powder, and chili powder. Cook this for 2 minutes, then turn off the heat.
7. When the squash is fork-tender, remove it from the oven and fill the holes with the bean and spinach mixture.
8. Serve warm.

Nutrition: Calories: 365 kcal, Fats: 34.6 g, Carbs: 16.7 g, Protein: 11.2 g

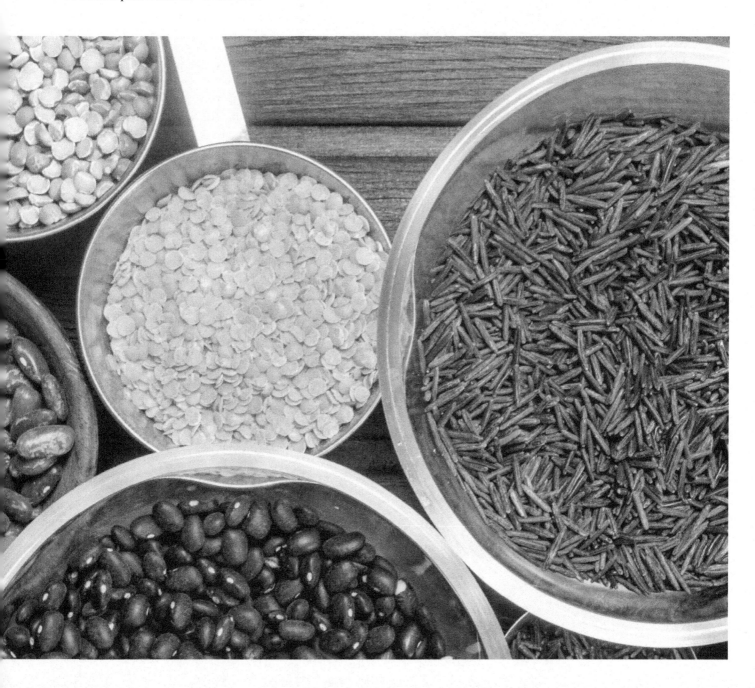

Chapter 7: Rice, Grains, and Legumes

33. Beluga Lentil and Vegetable Mélange

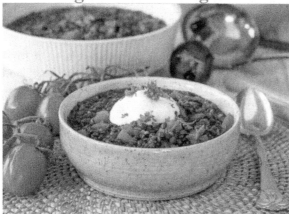

Preparation Time: 10 minutes, **Cooking Time:** 30 minutes, **Difficulty Level:** Moderate, **Servings:** 4

Ingredients:
- 3 Tbsp. olive oil
- 1 onion, minced
- 2 bell peppers, seeded and chopped
- 1 carrot, trimmed and chopped
- 1 parsnip, trimmed and chopped
- 1 tsp. ginger, minced
- 2 garlic cloves, minced
- Sea salt and ground black pepper, to taste
- 1 large-sized zucchini, diced
- 1 cup tomato sauce
- 1 cup vegetable broth
- 1 ½ cups beluga lentils, soaked overnight and drained
- 2 cups Swiss chard

Directions:
1. In a Dutch oven, heat the olive oil until sizzling. Now, sauté the onion, bell pepper, carrot, and parsnip, until they've softened.
2. Add in the ginger and garlic and continue sautéing for an additional 30 seconds.
3. Now, add in the salt, black pepper, zucchini, tomato sauce, vegetable broth, and lentils; let it simmer for about 20 minutes until everything is thoroughly cooked.
4. Add in the Swiss chard; cover and let it simmer for 5 minutes more.

Nutrition: Calories: 382 kcal, Fat: 9.3 g, Carbs: 59 g, Protein: 17.2 g

34. Vegan Chicken & Rice

Preparation Time: 15 minutes, **Cooking Time:** 3 hours and 30 minutes, **Difficulty Level:** Moderate, **Servings:** 4

Ingredients:
- 8 oz. Tofu
- Salt and pepper, to taste
- ½ tsp. ground coriander
- 2 tsp. ground cumin
- 17 oz. brown rice, cooked
- 30 oz. black beans
- 1 Tbsp. olive oil
- Pinch cayenne pepper
- 2 cups Pico De Gallo
- ¾ cup radish, sliced thinly
- 2 avocados, sliced

Directions:
1. Season the tofu with salt, pepper, coriander, and cumin.
2. Place in a slow cooker.
3. Pour in the stock.
4. Cook on low setting for 3 hours and 30 minutes.
5. Place the tofu on a cutting board.
6. Shred the tofu.
7. Toss the tofu shreds in the cooking liquid.
8. In bowls, serve the rice topped with the tofu and the rest of the ingredients.

Nutrition: Calories: 470 kcal, Fat: 17.0 g, Saturated Fat: 3.0 g, Sodium: 615 mg, Carbohydrates: 40.0 g, Fiber: 11.0 g, Sugar: 1.0 g, Protein: 40.0 g

35. Mango Sticky Rice

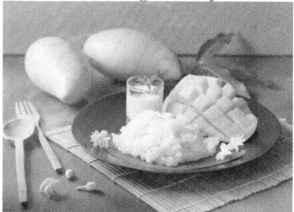

Preparation Time: 25 minutes, **Cooking Time:** 30 minutes, **Difficulty Level:** Moderate, **Servings:** 4

Ingredients:
- ½ Cup Sugar
- 1 Mango, Sliced
- 14 oz. Coconut Milk, Canned
- ½ Cup Basmati Rice

Directions:
1. Cook your rice per package instructions and add half of your sugar. When cooking your rice, substitute half of your water for half of your coconut milk.
2. Boil your remaining coconut milk in a saucepan with your remaining sugar.
3. Boil on high heat until it's thick, and then add in your mango slices.

Interesting Facts:
Mangos contain 50% of the daily Vitamin C you should consume, which aids in bone and immune health.

Nutrition: Calories: 577 kcal, Fat: 57.3 g, Carbs: 19.7 g, Fiber: 6.1 g, Protein: 5.7 g

36.   Rice Bowl with Edamame

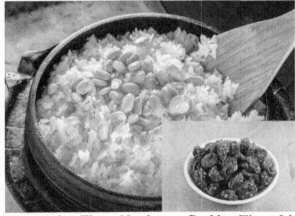

Preparation Time: 10 minutes, **Cooking Time:** 3 hours and 50 minutes, **Difficulty Level:** Hard, **Servings:** 4

Ingredients:
- 1 Tbsp. coconut oil, melted
- ¾ cup brown rice (uncooked)
- 1 cup wild rice (uncooked)
- Cooking spray
- 4 cups vegetable stock
- 8 oz. shelled edamame
- 1 onion, chopped
- Salt, to taste
- ½ cup dried cherries, sliced
- ½ cup pecans, toasted and sliced
- 1 Tbsp. red wine vinegar

Directions:
1. Add the rice and coconut oil in a slow cooker sprayed with oil. Pour in the stock and stir in the edamame and onions.
2. Season with salt. Seal the pot.
3. For 3 hours and 30 minutes, cook on high. Stir in the dried cherries.
4. Let sit for 5 minutes. Before serving, stir in the rest of the ingredients.

Nutrition: Calories: 381 kcal, Fat: 12.0 g 18%, Saturated Fat: 2.0 g, Sodium: 459 mg, Carbohydrates: 61.0 g, Fiber: 7.0 g, Sugar: 13.0 g, Protein: 12.0 g

37.   Instant Pot Millet Pilaf

Preparation Time: 20 minutes, **Cooking Time:** 11 minutes, **Difficulty Level:** Moderate, **Servings:** 4-5

Ingredients:
- 1 cup millet
- Cup apricot and shelled pistachios (roughly chopped)
- 1 lemon juice and zest
- 1 Tbsp. olive oil
- Cup parsley (fresh)

Directions:
1. Pour one and three-quarter cups of water into your instant pot. Place the millet and lid on the instant pot.
2. Adjust Time for 10 minutes on high pressure. When the Time has elapsed, release pressure naturally.
3. Remove the lid and add all other ingredients. Stir while adjusting the seasonings.
4. Serve and enjoy

Nutrition: Carbs: 33.3 g, Protein: 14.6 g, Fats: 26.6 g, Calories: 456 kcal

38.   Quinoa with Mixed Herbs

Preparation Time: 15 minutes, **Cooking Time:** 20 minutes, **Difficulty Level:** Moderate, **Servings:** 4

Ingredients:
- 1 cup quinoa, well-rinsed
- 2 cups vegetable broth
- Salt, to taste
- 2 garlic cloves, minced and divided
- ¼ cup chopped chives
- 2 Tbsp. finely chopped parsley
- 2 Tbsp. finely chopped basil
- 2 Tbsp. finely chopped mint
- 2 Tbsp. finely chopped soft sundried tomatoes

- 1 Tbsp. olive oil (optional)
- ½ tsp. lemon zest
- 1 Tbsp. fresh lemon juice
- 2 Tbsp. minced walnuts
- Salt and black pepper, to taste

Directions:
1. Combine the quinoa, vegetable broth, ¼ tsp. of salt, and half garlic in a medium pot. Boil the quinoa until it is tender and the liquid is absorbed (10-15 minutes).
2. Open the lid, fluff with a fork, and stir in the chives, parsley, basil, mint, tomatoes, olive oil, zest, lemon juice, and walnuts. Warm for 5 minutes.
3. Dish the food and serve warm.

Nutrition: Calories: 393 kcal, Fats: 17.1 g, Carbs: 31.9 g, Protein: 27.8 g

39. Black-Eyed Peas with Walnuts and Pomegranate

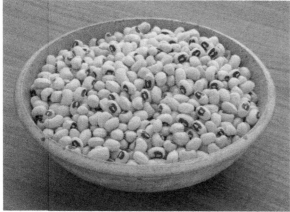

Preparation Time: 5 minutes, **Cooking Time:** None, **Difficulty Level:** Easy**, Servings:** 4 to 6

Ingredients:
- 3 Tbsp. extra-virgin olive oil
- 3 Tbsp. Dukkah
- 2 Tbsp. lemon juice
- 2 Tbsp. pomegranate molasses
- Salt and pepper, to taste
- 2 (15 oz.) cans black-eyed peas, rinsed
- ½ cup walnuts, toasted and chopped
- ½ cup pomegranate seeds
- ½ cup minced fresh parsley
- 4 scallions, sliced thin

Directions:
1. Whisk oil, 2 tablespoons of Dukkah, lemon juice, pomegranate molasses, ¼ tsp. salt, and ⅛ tsp. pepper together in a large bowl until smooth.

2. Add peas, walnuts, pomegranate seeds, parsley, and scallions and toss to combine. Season with salt and pepper to taste.
3. Sprinkle with the remaining 1 tablespoon of Dukkah and serve.

Nutrition: Calories: 348 kcal, Fat: 16.5 g, Carbs: 41.2 g, Protein: 7.2 g, Fiber: 5.3 g

40. Fresh Puttanesca with Quinoa

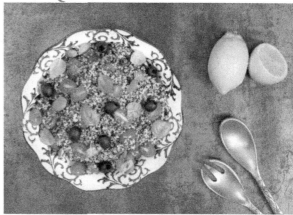

Preparation Time: 15 minutes, **Cooking Time:** 30 minutes, **Difficulty Level:** Moderate, **Servings:** 4

Ingredients:
- 1 cup brown quinoa
- 2 cups of water
- ⅛ tsp. salt
- 4 cups plum tomatoes, chopped
- 4 pitted green olives, sliced
- 4 pitted Kalamata olives, sliced
- 1 ½ Tbsp. capers, rinsed and drained
- 2 garlic cloves, minced
- 1 Tbsp. olive oil
- 1 Tbsp. chopped fresh parsley
- ¼ cup chopped fresh basil
- ⅛ tsp. red chili flakes

Directions:
1. Add the salt, water, and quinoa to a medium pot and cook covered over medium heat until tender and water is absorbed for about 10 to 15 minutes.
2. Meanwhile, mix the tomatoes, green olives, Kalamata olives, capers, garlic, olive oil, parsley, basil, and red chili flakes in a medium bowl. Allow sitting for 5 minutes.
3. Serve the Puttanesca with the quinoa.

Nutrition: Calories: 427 kcal, Fats: 7.1 g, Carbs: 88.2 g, Protein: 7.2 g

41. Brown Rice Salad

Preparation Time: 10 minutes, **Cooking Time:** 0 minutes, **Difficulty Level:** Easy, **Servings:** 4

Ingredients:
- 9 oz. brown rice, cooked
- 7 cups baby arugula
- 15 oz. canned garbanzo beans, drained and rinsed
- 4 oz. feta cheese, crumbled
- ¾ cup basil, chopped
- A pinch salt and black pepper
- 2 Tbsp. lemon juice
- ¼ tsp. lemon zest, grated
- ¼ cup olive oil

Directions:
1. In a salad bowl, combine the brown rice with the arugula, the beans, and the rest of the ingredients, toss and serve cold for breakfast.

Nutrition: Calories: 274 kcal, Fat: 5.4 g, Saturated Fat: 0.5 g, Carbohydrates: 57.3 g, Fiber: 13.3 g, Sugars: 33.8 g, Protein: 0.5 g

42. Bulgur and Garbanzo Pilaf

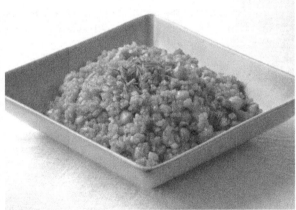

Preparation Time: 5 minutes, **Cooking Time:** 20 minutes, **Difficulty Level:** Moderate, **Servings:** 4

Ingredients:
- 3 Tbsp. extra-virgin olive oil
- 1 large onion, chopped
- 1 (16 oz.) can garbanzo beans, rinsed and drained
- 2 cups bulgur wheat #3, rinsed and drained
- 1½ tsp. salt
- ½ tsp. cinnamon
- 4 cups water

Directions:
1. In a large pot over medium heat, cook both the olive oil and onion for 5 minutes.

2. Add the garbanzo beans and cook for 5 minutes.
3. Add the bulgur, salt, cinnamon, and water and stir. Cover the pot, turn the heat to low, and cook for another 10 minutes.
4. When the cooking is done, fluff the pilaf with a fork. Cover and let sit for another 5 minutes.

Nutrition: Calories: 274 kcal, Fat: 5.4 g, Saturated Fat: 0.5 g, Carbohydrates: 57.3 g, Fiber: 13.3 g, Sugars: 33.8 g, Protein: 0.5 g

43. Chickpea Cakes

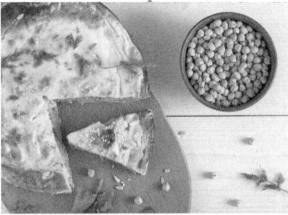

Preparation Time: 5 minutes, **Cooking Time:** 10 minutes, **Difficulty Level:** Hard, **Servings:** 4

Ingredients:
- 2 (15 oz.) cans chickpeas, rinsed
- ½ cup plain Greek yogurt
- 2 large eggs
- 6 Tbsp. extra-virgin olive oil
- 1 tsp. ground coriander
- ⅛ tsp. cayenne pepper
- ⅛ tsp. salt
- 1 cup panko breadcrumbs
- 2 scallions, sliced thin
- 3 Tbsp. minced fresh cilantro
- 1 shallot, minced
- 1 recipe Cucumber-Yogurt Sauce

Directions:
1. Pulse chickpeas in a food processor until coarsely ground, about 8 pulses. Whisk yogurt, eggs, 2 tablespoons of oil, coriander, cayenne, and salt together in a medium bowl. Gently stir in chickpeas, panko, scallions, cilantro, and shallot until just combined. Divide mixture into 6 equal portions and gently pack into 1-inch-thick patties.
2. Heat 2 tablespoons of oil in a 12-inch nonstick skillet over medium heat until shimmering. Carefully lay 3 patties in a skillet and cook until well browned and firm, 4 to 5 minutes per side.

3. Transfer cakes to a paper towel-lined plate and tent loosely with aluminum foil. Repeat with the remaining 2 tablespoons of oil and the remaining 3 patties. Serve with yogurt sauce.

Nutrition: Calories: 274 kcal, Fat: 5.4 g, Saturated Fat: 0.5 g, Carbohydrates: 57.3 g, Fiber: 13.3 g, Sugars: 33.8 g, Protein: 0.5 g

44. Confetti Couscous

Preparation Time: 5 minutes, **Cooking Time:** 20 minutes, **Difficulty Level:** Moderate, **Servings:** 4 to 6

Ingredients:
- 3 Tbsp. extra-virgin olive oil
- 1 large onion, chopped
- 2 carrots, chopped
- 1 cup fresh peas
- ½ cup golden raisins
- 1 tsp. salt
- 2 cups vegetable broth
- 2 cups couscous

Directions:
1. In a medium pot over medium heat, gently toss the olive oil, onions, carrots, peas, and raisins together and let cook for 5 minutes.
2. Add the salt and broth and stir to combine. Bring to a boil, and let ingredients boil for 5 minutes.
3. Add the couscous. Stir, turn the heat to low, cover, and let cook for 10 minutes. Fluff with a fork and serve.
4. Substitution tip: You can substitute the peas or carrots for other vegetables of your choice. Serve with fresh chopped parsley for extra flavor.

Nutrition: Calories: 274 kcal, Fat: 5.4 g, Saturated Fat: 0.5 g, Carbohydrates: 57.3 g, Fiber: 13.3 g, Sugars: 33.8 g, Protein: 0.5 g

45. Cranberry Beans with Fennel, Grapes, and Pine Nuts

Preparation Time: 5 minutes, **Cooking Time:** 1 Hour and 30 minutes, **Difficulty Level:** Hard, **Servings:** 4

Ingredients:
- Salt and pepper, to taste
- 1 lb. (2½ cups) dried cranberry beans, picked over and rinsed
- 3 Tbsp. extra-virgin olive oil
- ½ fennel bulb, 2 Tbsp. fronds chopped, stalks discarded, bulb cored and chopped
- 1 cup plus 2 Tbsp. red wine vinegar

- ½ cup sugar
- 1 tsp. fennel seeds
- 6 oz. seedless red grapes, halved (1 cup)
- ½ cup pine nuts, toasted

Directions:
1. Dissolve 3 tablespoons of salt in 4 quarts of cold water in a large container. Add beans and soak at room temperature for at least 8 hours or up to 24 hours.
2. Drain and rinse well. Bring beans, 4 quarts of water, and 1 tsp. salt to boil in a Dutch oven. Reduce to simmer and cook, occasionally stirring, until beans are tender, 1 to 1½ hours. Drain beans and set aside.
3. Wipe Dutch oven clean with paper towels. Heat oil in the now-empty pot over medium heat until it shimmers.
4. Add fennel, ¼ tsp. salt, and ¼ tsp. pepper and cook until softened, about 5 minutes. Stir in 1 cup vinegar, sugar, and fennel seeds until sugar is dissolved.
5. Bring to a simmer and cook until liquid is thickened to syrupy glaze and edges of fennel are beginning to brown, about 10 minutes.
6. Add beans to the vinegar-fennel mixture and toss to coat.
7. Transfer to a large bowl and let cool to room temperature. Add grapes, pine nuts, fennel fronds, and the remaining 2 tablespoons vinegar and toss to combine. Season with salt and pepper to taste and serve.

Nutrition: Calories: 274 kcal, Fat: 5.4 g, Saturated Fat: 0.5 g, Carbohydrates: 57.3 g, Fiber: 13.3 g, Sugars: 33.8 g, Protein: 0.5 g

46. Creamy Millet

Preparation Time: 10 minutes, **Cooking Time:** 15 minutes, **Difficulty Level:** Moderate, **Servings:** 4

Ingredients:

- 2 cups millet
- 1 cup almond milk, unsweetened
- 1 cup water
- 1 cup coconut milk, unsweetened
- 1 tsp. cinnamon
- ½ tsp. ground ginger
- ¼ tsp. salt
- 1 Tbsp. chia seeds
- 1 Tbsp. cashew butter
- 4 oz. Parmesan cheese, grated

Directions:

1. Combine the coconut milk, almond milk, and water in the saucepan.
2. Stir the liquid gently and add millet.
3. Mix carefully and close the lid.
4. Cook the millet on medium heat for 5 minutes.
5. Sprinkle the porridge with cinnamon, ground ginger, salt, and chia seeds.
6. Stir the mixture carefully with a spoon and continue to cook on medium heat for 5 minutes more.
7. Add the cashew butter and cook the millet for 5 minutes.
8. Remove the millet from the heat and transfer it to serving bowls.
9. Sprinkle the dish with the grated cheese.
10. Serve hot.

Nutrition: Calories: 274 kcal, Fat: 5.4 g, Saturated Fat: 0.5 g, Carbohydrates: 57.3 g, Fiber: 13.3 g, Sugars: 33.8 g, Protein: 0.5 g

47. Earthy Lentil and Rice Pilaf

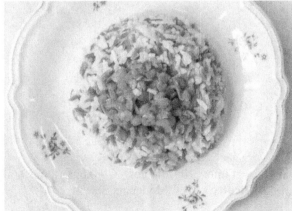

Preparation Time: 5 minutes, **Cooking Time:** 50 minutes, **Difficulty Level:** Moderate, **Servings:** 4

Ingredients:

- ¼ cup extra-virgin olive oil
- 1 large onion, chopped

- 6 cups water
- 1 tsp. ground cumin
- 1 tsp. salt
- 2 cups brown lentils, picked over and rinsed
- 1 cup basmati rice

Directions:

1. In a medium putting cook, the olive oil and onions for 7 to 10 minutes over medium heat until the edges are browned.
2. Turn the heat to high, add water, cumin, and salt, and boil the mixture for about 3 minutes.
3. Add the lentils and turn the heat to medium-low. Cover the pot and cook for 20 minutes, stirring occasionally.
4. Stir in the rice and cover; cook for an additional 20 minutes.
5. Fluff the rice with a fork and serve warm.

Nutrition:
Calories: 274 kcal, Fat: 5.4 g, Saturated Fat: 0.5 g, Carbohydrates: 57.3 g, Fiber: 13.3 g, Sugars: 33.8 g, Protein: 0.5 g

48. Easy and Hearty Shakshuka

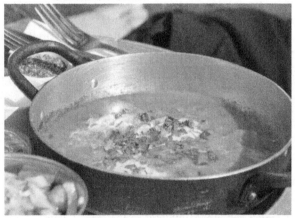

Preparation Time: 10 minutes, **Cooking Time:** 54 minutes, **Difficulty Level:** Moderate, **Servings:** 4

Ingredients:

- 2 Tbsp. olive oil
- 1 onion, chopped
- 2 bell peppers, chopped
- 1 Poblano pepper, chopped
- 2 cloves garlic, minced
- 2 tomatoes, pureed
- Sea salt and black pepper, to taste
- 1 tsp. dried basil
- 1 tsp. red pepper flakes
- 1 tsp. paprika
- 2 bay leaves

- 1 cup chickpeas, soaked overnight, rinsed, and drained
- 3 cups vegetable broth
- 2 Tbsp. fresh cilantro, roughly chopped

Directions:
1. Heat the olive oil in a saucepan over medium heat. Once hot, cook the onion, peppers, and garlic for about 4 minutes, until tender and aromatic.
2. Add the pureed tomato tomatoes, sea salt, black pepper, basil, red pepper, paprika, and bay leaves.
3. Turn the heat to a simmer and add in the chickpeas and vegetable broth. Cook for 45 minutes or until tender.
4. Taste and adjust seasonings. Spoon your Shakshuka into individual bowls and serve garnished with fresh cilantro.

Nutrition: Calories: 324 kcal, Fat: 11.2 g, Carbs: 42.2 g, Protein: 15.8 g

49.   Easy Red Lentil Salad

Preparation Time: 10 minutes, **Cooking Time:** 25 minutes, **Difficulty Level:** Easy, **Servings:** 4

Ingredients:
- ½ cup red lentils, soaked overnight and drained
- 1 ½ cups water
- 1 sprig rosemary
- 1 bay leaf
- 1 cup grape tomatoes, halved
- 1 cucumber, thinly sliced
- 1 bell pepper, thinly sliced
- 1 clove garlic, minced
- 1 onion, thinly sliced
- 2 Tbsp. fresh lime juice
- 4 Tbsp. olive oil
- Sea salt and ground black pepper, to taste

Directions:
1. Add the red lentils, water, rosemary, and bay leaf to a saucepan and bring to a boil over high heat. Then, turn the heat to a simmer and continue to cook for 20 minutes or until tender.
2. Place the lentils in a salad bowl and let them cool completely.
3. Add in the remaining ingredients and toss to combine well. Serve at room temperature or well-chilled.

Nutrition: Calories: 295 kcal, Fat: 18.8 g, Carbs: 25.2 g, Protein: 8.5 g

50.   Lemon Orzo with Fresh Herbs

Preparation Time: 10 minutes, **Cooking Time:** 10 minutes, **Difficulty Level:** Easy, **Servings:** 4

Ingredients:
- 2 cups Orzo
- ½ cup fresh parsley, finely chopped
- ½ cup fresh basil, finely chopped
- 2 Tbsp. lemon zest
- ½ cup extra-virgin olive oil
- ⅓ cup lemon juice
- 1 tsp. salt
- ½ tsp. freshly ground black pepper

Directions:
1. Bring a large pot of water to a boil. Add the orzo and cook for 7 minutes. Drain and rinse with cold water. Let the orzo sit in a strainer to drain and cool completely.
2. Once the orzo has cooled, put it in a large bowl and add the parsley, basil, and lemon zest.
3. In a small bowl, whisk together the olive oil, lemon juice, salt, and pepper. Add the dressing to the pasta and toss everything together. Serve at room temperature or chilled.

Nutrition: Calories: 212 kcal, Fats: 11.38 g, Carbs: 23.28 g, Proteins: 5.76 g

51.   Lentils and Bulgur with Caramelized Onions

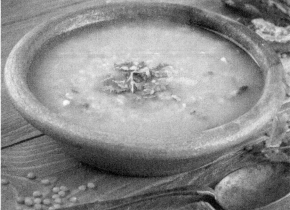

Preparation Time: 10 minutes, **Cooking Time:** 50 minutes, **Difficulty Level:** Moderate, **Servings:** 4

Ingredients:
- ½ cup extra-virgin olive oil
- 4 large onions, chopped
- 2 tsp. salt, divided
- 6 cups water
- 2 cups brown lentils, picked over and rinsed

- 1 tsp. freshly ground black pepper
- 1 cup bulgur wheat #3

Directions:
1. In a large pot over medium heat, cook and stir the olive oil, onions, and 1 tsp. of salt for 12 to 15 minutes, until the onions are medium brown/golden.
2. Put half of the cooked onions in a bowl.
3. Add the water, remaining 1 tsp. of salt, and lentils to the remaining onions. Stir. Cover and cook for 30 minutes.
4. Stir in the black pepper and bulgur, cover, and cook for 5 minutes. Fluff with a fork, cover, and let stand for another 5 minutes.
5. Spoon the lentils and bulgur onto a serving plate and top with the reserved onions. Serve warm.

Nutrition: Calories: 640 kcal, Fats: 18 g Carbs: 98 g, Proteins: 28.8 g

52. Mashed Fava Beans with Cumin and Garlic

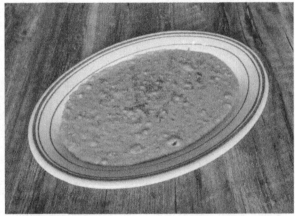

Preparation Time: 5 minutes, **Cooking Time:** 12 minutes, **Difficulty Level:** Moderate, **Servings:** 4

Ingredients:
- 4 garlic cloves, minced
- 1 Tbsp. extra-virgin olive oil, plus extra for serving
- 1 tsp. ground cumin
- 2 (15- oz.) cans fava beans
- 3 Tbsp. tahini
- 2 Tbsp. lemon juice, plus lemon wedges for serving
- Salt and pepper, to taste
- 1 tomato, cored and cut into ½-inch pieces
- 1 small onion, chopped fine
- 2 Tbsp. minced fresh parsley
- 2 hard-cooked large eggs, chopped

Directions:

1. Cook garlic, oil, and cumin in a medium saucepan over medium heat until fragrant, about 2 minutes. Stir in beans and their liquid and tahini. Bring to a simmer and cook until liquid thickens slightly 8 to 10 minutes.
2. Off heat, mash beans to a coarse consistency using a potato masher. Stir in lemon juice and 1 tsp. pepper. Season with salt and pepper to taste. Transfer to a serving dish, top with tomato, onion, parsley, and eggs, if using, and drizzle with extra oil. Serve with lemon wedges.

Nutrition: Calories: 616 kcal, Fats: 14 g, Carbs: 89 g Proteins: 3.6 g

53. Mediterranean-Style Chickpea Salad

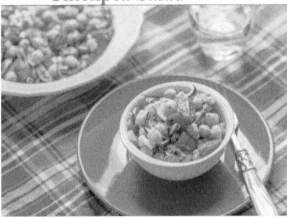

Preparation Time: 10 minutes, **Cooking Time:** 45 minutes, **Difficulty Level:** Moderate, **Servings:** 4

Ingredients:
- 2 cups chickpeas, soaked overnight, and drained
- 1 Persian cucumber, sliced
- 1 cup cherry tomatoes, halved
- 1 red bell pepper, seeded and sliced
- 1 green bell pepper, seeded and sliced
- 1 tsp. deli mustard
- 1 tsp. coriander seeds
- 1 tsp. jalapeno pepper, minced
- 1 Tbsp. fresh lemon juice
- 1 Tbsp. balsamic vinegar
- ¼ cup extra-virgin olive oil
- Sea salt and ground black pepper, to taste
- 2 Tbsp. fresh cilantro, chopped
- 2 Tbsp. Kalamata olives, pitted and sliced

Directions:
1. Place the chickpeas in a stockpot; cover the chickpeas with water by 2 inches. Bring it to a boil.
2. Immediately turn the heat to a simmer and continue to cook for about 40 minutes or until tender.

3. Transfer your chickpeas to a salad bowl. Add in the remaining ingredients and toss to combine well.

Nutrition: Calories: 468 kcal, Fat: 12.5 g, Carbs: 73 g, Protein: 21.8 g

54.   Mushroom Risotto

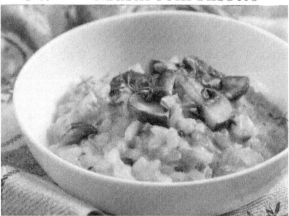

Preparation Time: 10 minutes, **Cooking Time:** 30 minutes, **Difficulty Level:** Moderate, **Servings:** 4

Ingredients:
- 6 cups vegetable broth
- 3 Tbsp. extra-virgin olive oil, divided
- 1- lb. cremini mushrooms, cleaned and sliced
- 1 medium onion, finely chopped
- 2 cloves garlic, minced
- 1½ cups Arborio rice
- 1 tsp. salt
- ½ cup freshly grated Parmesan cheese
- ½ tsp. freshly ground black pepper

Directions:
1. In a saucepan over medium heat, bring the broth to a low simmer.
2. In a large skillet over medium heat, cook 1 tablespoon olive oil and the sliced mushrooms for 5 to 7 minutes. Set cooked mushrooms aside.
3. In the same skillet over medium heat, add the 2 remaining tablespoons of olive oil, onion, and garlic. Cook for 3 minutes.
4. Add the rice, salt, and 1 cup of broth to the skillet. Stir the ingredients together and cook over low heat until most of the liquid is absorbed. Continue adding ½ cup of broth at a Time, stirring until it is absorbed. Repeat until all of the broth is used up.
5. With the final addition of broth, add the cooked mushrooms, Parmesan cheese, and black pepper. Cook for 2 more minutes.
6. Serve immediately.

Nutrition: Calories: 274 kcal, Fat: 5.4 g, Saturated Fat: 0.5 g, Carbohydrates: 57.3 g, Fiber: 13.3 g, Sugars: 33.8 g, Protein: 0.5 g

55.   Old-Fashioned Chili

Preparation Time: 10 minutes, **Cooking Time:** 1 hour & 40 minutes, **Difficulty Level:** Hard, **Servings:** 4

Ingredients:
- ¾ lb. red kidney beans, soaked overnight
- 2 Tbsp. olive oil
- 1 onion, chopped
- 2 bell peppers, chopped
- 1 red chili pepper, chopped
- 2 ribs celery, chopped
- 2 garlic cloves, minced
- 2 bay leaves
- 1 tsp. ground cumin
- 1 tsp. thyme, chopped
- 1 tsp. black peppercorns
- 20 oz. tomatoes, crushed
- 2 cups vegetable broth
- 1 tsp. smoked paprika
- Sea salt, to taste
- 2 Tbsp. fresh cilantro, chopped
- 1 avocado, pitted, peeled, and sliced

Directions:
1. Cover the soaked beans with a fresh change of cold water and bring to a boil. Let it boil for about 10 minutes. Turn the heat to a simmer and continue to cook for 50 to 55 minutes or until tender.
2. In a heavy-bottomed pot, heat the olive oil over medium heat. Once hot, sauté the onion, bell pepper, and celery.
3. Sauté the garlic, bay leaves, ground cumin, thyme, and black peppercorns for about 1 minute or so.
4. Add in the diced tomatoes, vegetable broth, paprika, salt, and cooked beans. Let it simmer, stirring periodically, for 25 to 30 minutes or until cooked through.
5. Serve garnished with fresh cilantro and avocado.

Nutrition: Calories: 514 kcal, Fat: 16.4 g, Carbs: 72 g, Protein: 25.8 g

56.   Orzo-Veggie Pilaf

Preparation Time: 20 minutes, **Cooking Time:** 10 minutes, **Difficulty Level:** Easy, **Servings:** 4

Ingredients:
- 2 cups orzo
- 1-pint (2 cups) cherry tomatoes, cut in half

- 1 cup Kalamata olives
- ½ cup fresh basil, finely chopped
- ½ cup extra-virgin olive oil
- ⅓ cup balsamic vinegar
- 1 tsp. salt
- ½ tsp. freshly ground black pepper

Directions:
1. Bring a large pot of water to a boil. Add the orzo and cook for 7 minutes. Drain and rinse the orzo with cold water in a strainer.
2. Once the orzo has cooled, put it in a large bowl. Add the tomatoes, olives, and basil.
3. In a small bowl, whisk together the olive oil, vinegar, salt, and pepper. Add this dressing to the pasta and toss everything together. Serve at room temperature or chilled.

Nutrition: Calories: 274 kcal, Fat: 5.4 g, Saturated Fat: 0.5 g, Carbohydrates: 57.3 g, Fiber: 13.3 g, Sugars: 33.8 g, Protein: 0.5 g

57. Overnight Berry Chia Oats

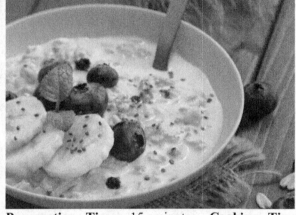

Preparation Time: 15 minutes, **Cooking Time:** 0 minute, **Difficulty Level:** Easy, **Servings:** 4

Ingredients:
- ½ cup Quaker Oats rolled oats
- ¼ cup chia seeds
- 1 cup milk or water
- Pinch of salt and cinnamon
- Maple syrup, or a different sweetener, to taste
- 1 cup frozen berries of choice, or smoothie leftovers

For the Toppings:
- Yogurt
- Berries

Directions:
1. In a jar with a lid, add the oats, seeds, milk, salt, and cinnamon, refrigerate overnight. On serving day, puree the berries in a blender.

2. Stir the oats, add in the berry puree, and top with yogurt and more berries, nuts, honey, or garnish of your choice. Enjoy!

Nutrition: Calories: 274 kcal, Fat: 5.4 g, Saturated Fat: 0.5 g, Carbohydrates: 57.3 g, Fiber: 13.3 g, Sugars: 33.8 g, Protein: 0.5 g

58. Rice Pudding

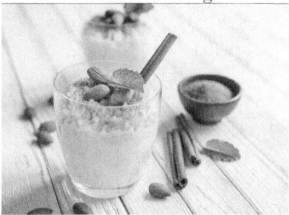

Preparation Time: 5 minutes, **Cooking Time:** 20 minutes, **Difficulty Level:** Moderate, **Servings:** 4

Ingredients:
- 1 cup brown rice
- 2 cups coconut milk, unsweetened
- 1 tsp. cinnamon
- 1 tsp. ginger
- ⅓ tsp. thyme
- ⅓ cup almonds
- 2 Tbsp. honey
- 1 tsp. lemon zest

Directions:
1. Pour the coconut milk into a saucepan and heat over medium.
2. Add the brown rice and stir the mixture carefully.
3. Close the lid and cook the brown rice over medium heat for 10 minutes.
4. Meanwhile, crush the almonds and combine them with lemon zest, thyme, ginger, and cinnamon.
5. Sprinkle the brown rice with the almond mixture and stir it carefully.
6. Close the lid and cook the dish for 5 minutes.
7. When the pudding is cooked, remove it from the saucepan and transfer it to a big bowl.
8. Add the honey and stir the pudding.
9. Serve it immediately.

Nutrition: Calories: 379 kcal, Fat: 5.0 g, Carbs: 6.0 g Fiber: 2.0 g, Protein: 4.0 g

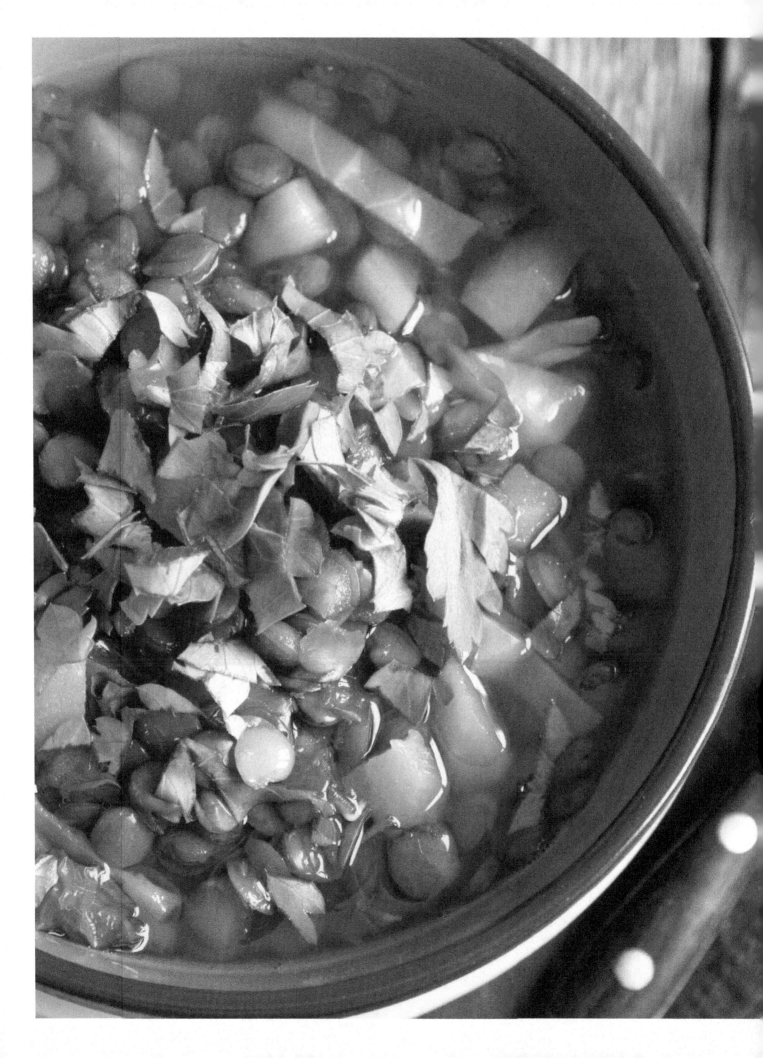

Chapter 8: Soups and Stews

62. Bean Stew

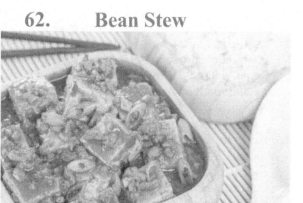

Preparation Time: 20 minutes, **Cooking Time:** 35 minutes, **Difficulty Level:** Moderate, **Servings:** 4

Ingredients:
- 1 kg fresh beans
- 2 beautiful onions
- 200 to 400 g smoked tofu (depending on appetite)
- 5 tsp.. oil neutral taste
- 2-3 tsp.. chopped fresh herbs
- 10 cl of water or vegetable broth
- Salt and pepper, to taste

Directions:
1. Shell the beans. Peel and finely chop the onions.
2. Cut the smoked tofu into cubes (half a centimeter per side). Heat the oil in a sauté pan. Add the onions, sauté gently, stirring. Add the smoked tofu and mix for 5 minutes.

3. Finally, add the beans and the chopped fresh herbs chosen. Mix. Salt and pepper. Moisten water or broth.
4. Simmer for 20 minutes, covered, stirring occasionally. Serve hot.

Nutrition: Calories: 206 kcal, Fiber: 15.0 g, Protein: 31.0 g

63. Sweet Chickpea and Mushroom Stew

Preparation Time: 10 minutes, **Cooking Time:** 8 minutes, **Difficulty Level:** Easy, **Servings:** 4

Ingredients:
- ½ Tbsp. button mushrooms, chopped
- 1 cup chickpeas, cooked

- 2 carrots, chopped
- 2 garlic cloves, crushed
- 4 cherry tomatoes
- 1 onion, peeled and chopped
- A handful of string beans, trimmed
- 1 apple, cut into 1-inch cubes
- ½ cup raisins
- A handful of fresh mint
- 1 tsp. ginger, grated
- ½ cup orange juice, squeezed
- ½ tsp. salt

Directions:
1. Place all ingredients in your instant pot. Pour enough water to cover completely.
2. Cook on high pressure for 8 minutes. Quick-release the pressure over 10 minutes
3. Serve and enjoy!

Nutrition: Calories: 577 kcal, Fat: 57.3 g, Carbs: 19.7 g, Fiber: 6.1 g, Protein: 5.7 g

64. Traditional Tuscan Bean Stew (Ribollita)

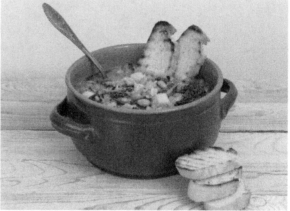

Preparation Time: 10 minutes, **Cooking Time:** 22 minutes, **Difficulty Level:** Moderate, **Servings:** 4

Ingredients:
- 3 Tbsp. olive oil
- 1 medium leek, chopped
- 1 celery with leaves, chopped
- 1 zucchini, diced
- 1 Italian pepper, sliced
- 3 garlic cloves, crushed
- 2 bay leaves
- Kosher salt and ground black pepper, to taste
- 1 tsp. cayenne pepper
- 1 (28-oz.) can tomatoes, crushed

- 2 cups vegetable broth
- 2 (15-oz.) cans Great Northern beans, drained
- 2 cups Lacinato kale, torn into pieces
- 1 cup crostini

Directions:
1. In a heavy-bottomed pot, heat the olive oil over medium heat. Once hot, sauté the leek, celery, zucchini, and pepper for about 4 minutes.
2. Sauté the garlic and bay leaves for about 1 minute or so.
3. Add in the spices, tomatoes, broth, and canned beans. Let it simmer, occasionally stirring, for about 15 minutes or until cooked through.
4. Add in the Lacinato kale and continue simmering, occasionally stirring, for 4 minutes.
5. Serve garnished with crostini.

Nutrition: Calories: 379 kcal, Fat: 5.0 g, Carbs: 6.0 g, Fiber: 2.0 g, Protein: 4.0 g

65. Anasazi Bean and Vegetable Stew

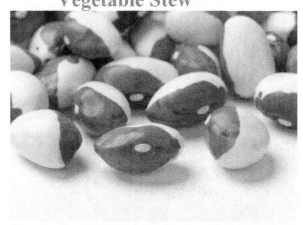

Preparation Time: 10 minutes, **Cooking Time:** 20 minutes, **Difficulty Level:** Moderate, **Servings:** 4

Ingredients:
- 1 cup Anasazi beans, soaked overnight, and drained
- 3 cups roasted vegetable broth
- 1 bay laurel
- 1 thyme sprig, chopped
- 1 rosemary sprig, chopped
- 3 Tbsp. olive oil
- 1 large onion, chopped
- 2 celery stalks, chopped
- 2 carrots, chopped
- 2 bell peppers, seeded and chopped
- Sea salt and ground black pepper, to taste
- 1 green chili pepper, seeded and chopped
- 2 garlic cloves, minced
- 1 tsp. cayenne pepper

- 1 tsp. paprika

Directions:
1. In a saucepan, bring the Anasazi beans and broth to a boil. Once boiling, turn the heat to a simmer. Add the bay laurel, thyme, and rosemary; let it cook for about 50 minutes or until tender.
2. Meanwhile, in a heavy-bottomed pot, heat the olive oil over medium-high heat. Now, sauté the onion, celery, carrots, and peppers for about 4 minutes until tender.
3. Add in the garlic and continue to sauté for 30 seconds more or until aromatic.
4. Add the sautéed mixture to the cooked beans. Season with salt, black pepper, cayenne pepper, and paprika.
5. Continue to simmer, stirring periodically, for 10 minutes more or until everything is cooked through.

Nutrition: Calories: 444 kcal, Fat: 15.8 g, Carbs: 58.2 g, Protein: 20.2 g

66. Cauliflower Curry Soup

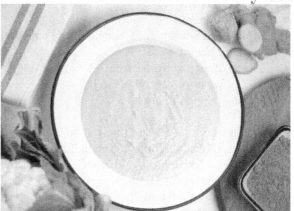

Preparation Time: 10 minutes, **Cooking Time:** 55 minutes, **Difficulty Level:** Moderate, **Servings:** 4

Ingredients:
- 1 large cauliflower head, chopped
- 4 Tbsp. coconut oil, divided
- 1 medium yellow onion, diced
- 3 Tbsp. Thai red curry paste
- ½ tsp. Seville orange zest
- ½ cup unoaked white wine
- 1 ½ cups vegetable stock
- 1 can (14 oz.) light coconut milk
- 1 to 3 tsp. rice vinegar
- Celtic sea salt, iodine-free, to taste
- Freshly ground black pepper, to taste
- 1 Tbsp. chopped fresh basil
- Nuts to garnish

Directions:

1. Preheat oven to 400F. Add cauliflower with coconut oil in a bowl. Spread it on a large baking sheet. Bake for about 25 to 30 minutes. Melt a tablespoon of coconut oil in a Dutch oven.
2. Add onion with a dash of salt to sauté for 3 minutes. Stir in curry paste and Seville orange zest. Mix well, then add wine and cook until it is completely absorbed. Add roasted cauliflower, coconut milk, and vegetable stock.
3. Let it cook for 10 minutes on a low simmer. Puree the soup using a handheld blender after cooling for 5 minutes. Adjust seasoning with salt and pepper. Garnish with basil and nuts.

Nutrition: Calories: 338 kcal, Fat: 3.8 g, Protein: 15.4 g

67. Dry Belly Soup Recipe with Cabbage

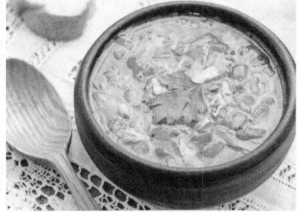

Preparation Time: 15 minutes, **Cooking Time:** 35 minutes, **Difficulty Level:** Moderate, **Servings:** 4

Ingredients:

- 4 chopped carrot
- 4 chopped turnip greens
- 8 tomatoes chopped without seeds
- 2 cups chopped cabbage into strips
- 4 oz. of the pod
- 8 cabbage leaves chopped into strips
- 4 chopped onion
- 4 Tbsp. olive oil
- Salt to taste

Directions:

1. Heat the olive oil in a pan. Sauté the onion and garlic in a pan. When golden, place the carrot and turnip, pour 500 ml of water, and cook for 20 minutes.
2. Add the remaining ingredients, add more water if necessary and bring to a boil for 10 minutes. Set seasonings and serve!

Nutrition: Calories:366 kcal, Fiber: 17.9 g, Protein: 18.5 g

68. Greek Vegetable Soup

Preparation Time: 55 minutes, **Cooking Time:** 20 minutes, **Difficulty Level:** Hard, **Servings:** 4

Ingredients:

- 3 Tbsp. of olive oil
- 1 onion, chopped
- 1 garlic clove, minced
- 3 cups of cabbage, shredded
- 2 medium carrots, chopped
- 2 celery sticks, chopped
- 2 cups cooked chickpeas
- 4 cups vegetable broth
- 15- oz. fire-roasted tomatoes, diced
- Salt and pepper, to taste

Directions:

1. Add olive oil to the instant pot and set to medium heat sauté.
2. Add the onions and cook until soft. Add garlic and cabbage and cook for another 5 minutes. When the cabbage softens, add the carrots, celery, and chickpeas. Stir everything to combine and cook for 5 minutes longer
3. Add the broth and canned tomatoes, then season with salt and pepper.
4. Press cancel to end sauté mode and cover the pot with the lid set to sealing mode.
5. Set to soup mode and adjust the Time to 10 minutes.
6. After completion, release the pressure manually and serve immediately.
7. You may garnish the soup with parsley, feta, or anything you like on soup.

Nutrition: Calories: 144 kcal, Fat: 7.0 g, Protein: 5.0 g, Carbohydrates: 18.0 g, Fiber: 3.0 g, Sugar: 0 g

69. Instant Pot Mediterranean Lentil and Collard Soup

Preparation Time: 20 minutes, **Cooking Time:** 22 minutes, **Difficulty Level:** Hard, **Servings:** 4

Ingredients:

- 2 Tbsp. extra-virgin olive oil
- 1 medium yellow onion, chopped
- 2 medium celery sticks, diced
- 3 garlic cloves, minced
- 2 tsp. ground cumin
- 1 tsp. ground turmeric
- 4 cups low-sodium vegetable broth

- 1 ¼ cup water
- 1 ½ cups dry brown lentils, rinsed in water
- 2 carrots, peeled and diced
- 1 bay leaf
- 1 tsp. Himalayan salt
- ½ tsp. ground black pepper
- 3 collard leaves, cut into strips
- 1 tsp. lemon juice

Directions:
1. **Set the instant** pot to sauté, add the olive oil, heat, and add onions and celery. Stir often for 5 minutes. Turn the instant pot off.
2. Stir in the garlic, cumin, and turmeric until combined.
3. Add broth, water, lentils, carrots, bay leaf, salt, and pepper. Lock the lid and close the valve. Set to manual and cook on high pressure for 13 minutes.
4. After completion, quickly release the pressure, carefully remove the lid and stir in collards and lemon juice.
5. Close the lid and set to manual and cook for 2 more minutes on high. Quick-release the pressure, open the lid, and it's ready to serve.

Nutrition: Calories: 144 kcal, Fat: 7.0 g, Protein: 5.0 g, Carbohydrates: 18.0 g, Fiber: 3.0 g, Sugar: 0 g

70.   Kale Soup

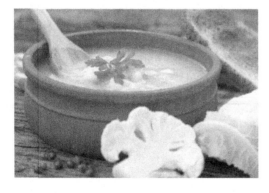

Preparation Time: 10 minutes, **Cooking Time:** 30 minutes, **Difficulty Level:** Moderate, **Servings:** 4

Ingredients:
- 2 Tbsp. olive oil
- ½ piece white onion, fileted
- 1 celery stick cut into cubes
- 1 cup chopped pore
- 1 Tbsp. finely chopped garlic
- 1 cup sliced mushrooms
- 1 cup mushroom, fileted
- 2 cups kale

- ½ piece fennel the bulb into sticks
- 6 cups beef broth
- 1 pinch salt
- 1 pinch pepper
- ¼ cup almond

Directions:
1. **Preheat a medium** deep pot at medium heat, cook olive oil, onion, and celery, add the pork, mushroom, and garlic until it releases the juice, put in kale with the fennel, and cook for 5 more minutes.
2. Pour the beef broth and season well. Cook, covering it to prevent it from evaporating. Sprinkle a little fresh kale and sliced almonds.

Nutrition: Calories: 507 kcal, Carbohydrates: 65.6 g, Proteins: 35.8 g

71.   Lentil Soup

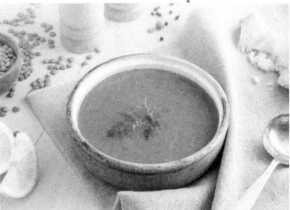

Preparation Time: 20 minutes, **Cooking Time:** 15 minutes, **Difficulty Level:** Easy, **Servings:** 4

Ingredients:
- ½ cup red lentil
- 3 cups vegetable broth
- 1 onion, chopped
- 2 cloves garlic, chopped
- Dried herb mixture, ½ tsp. of each (mint, parsley, sumac, cumin, coriander)

Directions:
1. Select the Sauté setting in the instant pot. Add 2 tablespoons of olive oil and the onion,, and cook for 3 minutes.
2. Then add garlic and herb mixture and cook for 2 minutes. Stir frequently.
3. Add lentils and broth, and then season with salt and pepper.
4. Close the lid and press manual mode. Cook for 8 minutes on High pressure.
5. Release the pressure naturally. Serve and enjoy!

Nutrition: Calories: 144 kcal, Fat: 7.0 g, Protein: 5.0 g, Carbohydrates: 18.0 g, Fiber: 3.0 g, Sugar: 0 g

72.   Melon Gazpacho

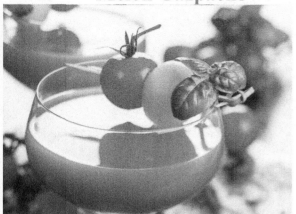

Preparation Time: 10 minutes, **Cooking Time:** 0 minute, **Difficulty Level:** Easy, **Servings:** 4

Ingredients:
- 1 lb. cantaloupe, peeled, chopped
- 1 Tbsp. avocado oil
- 1 red onion, diced
- ¼ cup of water
- 1 tsp. dried basil

Directions:
1. Incorporate all ingredients in the blender until smooth.
2. Pour the cooked gazpacho into the serving bowls.

Nutrition: Calories: 210 kcal, Fats: 8.19 g, Carbs: 19.72 g, Proteins: 1.22 g

73.   Peanut Stew

Preparation Time: 10 minutes, **Cooking Time:** 45 minutes, **Difficulty Level:** Moderate, **Servings:** 4

Ingredients:
- ¼ cup red lentils
- 2 medium sweet potatoes, peeled, cubed
- 1 medium white onion, peeled, diced
- 1 cup kale, chopped
- 2 tomatoes, diced
- ¼ cup chopped green onion
- 1 tsp. minced garlic
- 1 in. ginger, grated
- 2 Tbsp. toasted peanuts
- ¼ tsp. ground black pepper
- 1 tsp. ground cumin
- ½ tsp. turmeric
- ⅛ tsp. cayenne pepper
- 1 Tbsp. peanut butter
- 1 ½ cups vegetable broth

- 2 tsp. coconut oil

Directions:
1. Take a medium pot, place it on medium heat, add oil, add onions, and cook for 5 minutes when it melts.
2. Then stir in ginger and garlic, cook for 2 minutes until fragrant, add lentils and potatoes along with all the spices, and stir until mixed.
3. Stir in tomatoes, pour in the broth, bring the mixture to boil, switch heat to the low level, and simmer for 30 minutes until cooked.
4. Then, stir in peanut butter until incorporated and then puree by using an immersion blender until half-pureed.
5. Return stew over low heat, stir in kale, cook for 5 minutes until its leaves wilts, and then season with black pepper and salt.
6. Garnish the stew with peanuts and green onions, and then serve.

Nutrition: Calories: 401 kcal, Fat: 6.7 g, Carbs: 77.3 g, Protein: 10.8 g, Fiber: 16.0 g

74.   Pumpkin Soup

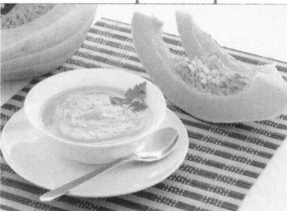

Preparation Time: 30 minutes, **Cooking Time:** 8 minutes, **Difficulty Level:** Easy, **Servings:** 4

Ingredients:
- 30 oz. pumpkin puree
- 1/4 chicken stock
- 1 onion, chopped
- 2 cups sweet potato, chopped
- 1 tsp. garlic powder

Directions:
1. Add all ingredients into your instant pot. Close the pot and press the Manual.
2. Cook for 8 minutes on High pressure and release the pressure naturally.
3. Then transfer it to your blender and blend until smooth. Season with salt and pepper.
4. Serve and enjoy!

Nutrition: Calories: 144 kcal, Fat: 7.0 g, Protein: 5.0 g, Carbohydrates: 18.0 g, Fiber: 3.0 g, Sugar: 0 g

75.   Simple Veggie Stew

Preparation Time: 40 minutes, **Cooking Time:** 22 minutes, **Difficulty Level:** Moderate, **Servings:** 4

Ingredients:
- 1 package mixed vegetables, frozen
- 4 cups vegetable broth
- 1 onion, minced
- 20 oz. tomato sauce
- 2 tsp. Italian seasoning

Directions:
1. Set the Instant pot to Sauté mode. Add 1 tablespoon of olive oil.
2. Cook onion for 1 minute. Add frozen vegetables and cook for 3 to 5 minutes, and then add the remaining ingredients.
3. Cover the pot and press Manual, and cook for 15 minutes on High pressure.
4. Release the pressure naturally and season with salt and pepper.
5. Serve and enjoy!

Nutrition: Calories: 144 kcal, Fat: 7.0 g, Protein: 5.0 g, Carbohydrates: 18.0 g, Fiber: 3.0 g, Sugar: 0 g

76.   Soup of Noodles with Vegetables

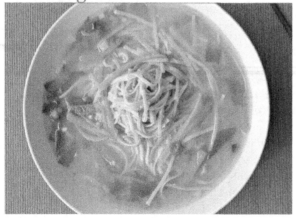

Preparation Time: 20 minutes, **Cooking Time:** 15 minutes, **Difficulty Level:** Moderate, **Servings:** 4

Ingredients:
- 2 lt. water
- 150g organic buckwheat noodles
- 2 garlic cloves
- 1 laminated tender onion
- 1 laminated leek
- 1 carrot cut in julienne
- 5 or 6 laminated mushrooms
- 1 trunk of celery, cut into thin slices
- ½ red pepper
- ½ green pepper
- 1 Tbsp.. fresh ginger
- 1 strip wakame seaweed
- 1 pinch sea salt
- Ground black pepper, to taste
- Extra virgin olive oil
- Soy sauce
- Parsley and chopped fresh chives, sprinkled

Directions:
1. Heat a tablespoon of oil in a pot with a lid and sauté the garlic, onion, and leek over medium heat.
2. Add the carrot, mushrooms, celery, red and green pepper cut into thin strips, the freshly grated ginger, and the seaweed. Cover and sauté for 3 to 4 minutes with the pot covered. If necessary, add some tablespoons of water to facilitate cooking.
3. Add salt, cover with water and boil on low heat for about 5 minutes. Bring two liters of boiling water to a separate pot and boil the noodles (follow the package instructions).
4. Drain, immediately pour a small number of noodles into a bowl and add the broth with the vegetables.
5. Season with a string of soy sauce, sprinkle with the herbs and dress with a string of olive oil. Serves hot.

Nutrition: Calories: 159 kcal, Fat:3.8 g, Protein: 5.8 g

77.   Spanish Chickpea and Sweet Potato Stew

Preparation Time: 5 minutes, **Cooking Time:** 35 minutes, **Difficulty Level:** Moderate, **Servings:** 4

Ingredients:
- 14 oz. cooked chickpeas
- 1 small sweet potato, peeled, cut into ½-inch cubes
- 1 medium red onion, sliced
- 3 oz. baby spinach
- 14 oz. crushed tomatoes
- 2 tsp. minced garlic
- 1 tsp. salt
- 1 ½ tsp. ground cumin
- 2 tsp. harissa paste
- 2 tsp. maple syrup
- ½ tsp. ground black pepper
- 2 tsp. sugar

- 1 Tbsp. olive oil
- ½ cup vegetable stock
- 2 Tbsp. chopped parsley
- 1 oz. slivered almonds, toasted
- Brown rice, cooked, for serving

Directions:
1. Take a large saucepan, place it over low heat, add oil, and when hot, add onion and garlic; cook for 5 minutes.
2. Then add sweet potatoes, season with cumin, stir in the harissa paste and cook for 2 minutes until toasted.
3. Switch heat to medium-low level, add tomatoes and chickpeas, pour in vegetable stock, stir in maple syrup and sugar and simmer for 25 minutes until potatoes have softened, stirring every 10 minutes.
4. Then add spinach, cook for 1 minute until its leaves have wilted, and season with salt and black pepper.
5. When done, distribute cooked rice between bowls, top with stew, garnish with parsley and almonds and serve.

Nutrition: Calories: 348 kcal, Fat: 16.5 g, Carbs: 41.2 g, Protein: 7.2 g, Fiber: 5.3 g

78.   Stewed Kidney Bean

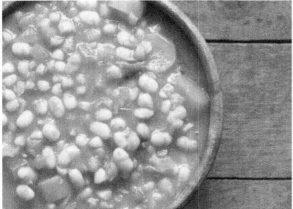

Preparation Time: 10 minutes, **Cooking Time:** 13 minutes, **Difficulty Level:** Moderate, **Servings:** 4

Ingredients:
- 6 oz. red beans, cooked
- 2 cups vegetable broth
- 1 onion, peeled and chopped
- 2 Tbsp. tomato paste
- 1 bay leaf
- 3 Tbsp. olive oil
- 2 carrots, chopped
- 2 celery stalks
- 1 tsp. salt

- Parsley, a handful

Directions:
1. Warm oil on Sauté mode and stir-fry onions for 3 minutes.
2. Add celery and carrots and cook for 5 minutes more. Add 1 tablespoon broth, beans, bay leaf, tomato paste, parsley, salt. Stir in 1 tablespoon flour and add the remaining broth.
3. Close the lid and cook on High pressure for 5 minutes. Quick-release the pressure over 10 minutes.
4. Add fresh parsley on top. Serve and enjoy!

Nutrition: Calories: 348 kcal, Fat: 16.5 g, Carbs: 41.2 g, Protein: 7.2 g, Fiber: 5.3 g

79.   Sweet Potato soup

Preparation Time: 15 minutes, **Cooking Time:** 35 minutes, **Difficulty Level:** Moderate, **Servings:** 4

Ingredients:
- 1 Tbsp. olive oil
- 2 garlic cloves, minced
- 1 medium chopped onion
- 3 tomatoes skinless and chopped seeds
- 2 chopped zucchinis
- 1 medium sweet potato chopped
- 2 cups chopped spinach
- Chopped parsley, to taste
- 1 lt. water
- Salt, to taste

Directions:
1. Inside a saucepan, heat the olive oil and then sauté the garlic, onion, and tomato. Add zucchini, peeled and chopped sweet potatoes, and spinach and cook for 5 minutes.
2. Add water, salt and cook until tender. Wait for the soup to simmer and beat in the blender until you get a creamy soup.
3. Return to the pot to heat, season seasoning if necessary, and serve with fresh parsley.

Nutrition: Calories: 133 kcal, Protein: 3.2 g, Fat: 5.3 g

80. Tomato and Garlic Soup

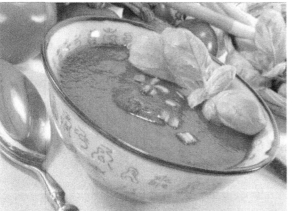

Preparation Time: 40 minutes, **Cooking Time:** 20 minutes, **Difficulty Level:** Moderate, **Servings:** 4

Ingredients:
- ½ liter water
- 1 purple onion
- 8-10 garlic cloves, rolled
- 1 kilo ripe tomatoes, without skin
- 2 or 3 bay leaves
- 1 pinch cayenne pepper
- 1 pinch black pepper
- Sea salt, to taste
- 1 tsp.. Provencal herbs
- 1 pinch cumin
- Extra virgin olive oil

Directions:
1. In a pot, sauté the onion and garlic in 1 tablespoon of olive oil. Remove often, so they do not burn. Blanch the tomatoes into boiling water, remove the skin, and, if you prefer, also the seeds.
2. Add to the pot the tomatoes cut in quarters and the rest of the ingredients. Remove and cook over low heat for 10 minutes and with the pot covered until the tomato acquires a slightly orange tone.
3. Add the water, and boil for about 10 minutes. Remove the bay leaves and crush them until you get a light texture. If necessary, add more water and rectify salt.
4. Serve the hot soup dressed with a strand of extra virgin olive oil and sprinkled with cumin.

Nutrition: Calories: 81.3 kcal, Fat:2.1 g, Protein: 31 g

81. Vegetables Soup

Preparation Time: 35 minutes, **Cooking Time:** 1 hour and 40 minutes, **Difficulty Level:** Hard, **Servings:** 4

Ingredients:
- 2 carrots
- 1 onion

- 4 shallots
- 1 white leek
- 1 celery branch
- 50 g celeriac
- ½ fennel
- 1 stick of lemongrass
- ½ bird's eye chili
- 25 g fresh ginger
- 3 garlic cloves
- 2 Tbsp. olive oil
- ½ tsp. ground black pepper
- ½ Tbsp. coarse salt
- 4 cloves
- 1-star anise

Directions:
1. Peel the vegetables. Cut the onion into quarters and then prick the cloves. Chop the shallots. Cut the carrots and celery stalks into sections. Cut the leek and ginger into slices. Slice the fennel. Coarsely chop the garlic cloves.
2. Cut the lemongrass in half lengthwise. Remove the seeds from the bird's eye pepper. Sweat all the ingredients in a saucepan with a little olive oil without letting them color. Add 2.5 l of water and simmer over low heat for 1 hour and 30 minutes while foaming from Time to Time to remove the impurities.
3. Remove from the heat, let stand for 30 minutes, then filter the broth using a fine strainer without squeezing the filling. You can keep this broth for 2 days in the refrigerator.

Nutrition: Calories:201 kcal,Protein: 60.0 g, Fiber: 31.0 g

82. Vegetarian Irish Stew

Preparation Time: 5 minutes, **Cooking Time:** 38 minutes, **Difficulty Level:** Moderate, **Servings:** 4

Ingredients:
- 1 cup textured vegetable protein, chunks
- ½ cup split red lentils
- 2 medium onions, peeled, sliced
- 1 cup sliced parsnip
- 2 cups sliced mushrooms
- 1 cup diced celery,
- ¼ cup flour
- 4 cups vegetable stock
- 1 cup rutabaga
- 1 bay leaf
- ½ cup fresh parsley
- 1 tsp. sugar
- ¼ tsp. ground black pepper
- ¼ cup soy sauce
- ¼ tsp. thyme
- 2 tsp. marmite
- ¼ tsp. rosemary

- ⅔ tsp. salt
- ¼ tsp. marjoram

Directions:
1. Take a large soup pot, place it over medium heat, add oil and when it gets hot, add the onions. Let it cook for 5 minutes or until softened.
2. Then, switch heat to the low level, sprinkle with flour, stir well, add remaining ingredients, stir until combined, and simmer for 30 minutes until vegetables have cooked.
3. When done, season the stew with salt and black pepper and then serve.

Nutrition: Calories: 270 kcal, Fat: 1.1 g, Carbs: 47.39 g, Protein: 20.15 g, Fiber: 7.5 g

83. Zucchini Turnip Soup

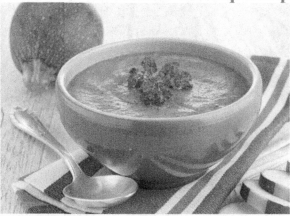

Preparation Time: 10 minutes, **Cooking Time:** 30 minutes, **Difficulty Level:** Moderate, **Servings:** 4

Ingredients:
- 1 Tbsp. coconut oil
- 2 cups yellow onion, chopped
- 2 chive cloves, minced
- 1 Tbsp. fresh ginger, minced
- 2 Tbsp. red curry paste
- 4 cups low-sodium vegetable broth
- 3 cups diced zucchinis, peeled
- 3 cups turnips, peeled and diced
- Celtic sea salt, iodine-free, to taste
- Freshly ground black pepper, to taste
- ¼ tsp. cayenne pepper

Directions:
1. Sauté chive, onion, and ginger in a greased pan for 5 to 6 minutes. Stir in curry paste and broth.
2. Mix well, then add zucchinis, salt, and turnips. Boil the soup on high heat. Cover the pot. Cook for 15 to 20 minutes. Blend this soup in a blender in batches until smooth.
3. Adjust seasoning with salt and pepper. Divide the soup into the serving bowl.

4. Serve warm.

Nutrition: Calories: 338 kcal, Fat: 3.8 g, Protein: 15.4 g

84. Arugula Pasta Soup

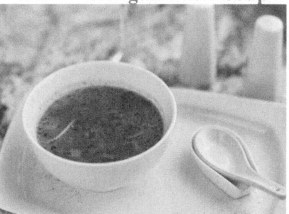

Preparation Time: 15 minutes, **Cooking Time:** 8 minutes, **Difficulty Level:** Moderate, **Servings:** 4

Ingredients:
- 7 oz. chickpeas, rinsed
- 4 eggs, lightly beaten
- 2 Tbsp.. lemon juice
- 3 cups arugula, chopped
- 6 Tbsp.. parmesan cheese
- 6 cups chicken broth
- 1 pinch nutmeg
- 1 bunch scallions, sliced (greens and whites sliced separately)
- 1 ⅓ cups whole-wheat pasta shells
- 2 cups water
- Ground black pepper, to taste

Directions:
1. Combine the pasta, scallion whites, chickpeas, water, broth, and nutmeg in a cooking pot or deep saucepan.
2. Heat the mixture, cover, and bring to a boil.
3. Take off the lid and simmer the mixture for about 4 minutes before adding the arugula. Then cook until it is wilted.
4. Mix in the eggs and season with black pepper and salt.
5. Mix in the lemon juice and scallion greens. Top with the parmesan cheese; serve warm.

Nutrition: Calories: 577 kcal, Fat: 57.3 g, Carbs: 19.7 g, Fiber: 6.1 g, Protein: 5.7 g

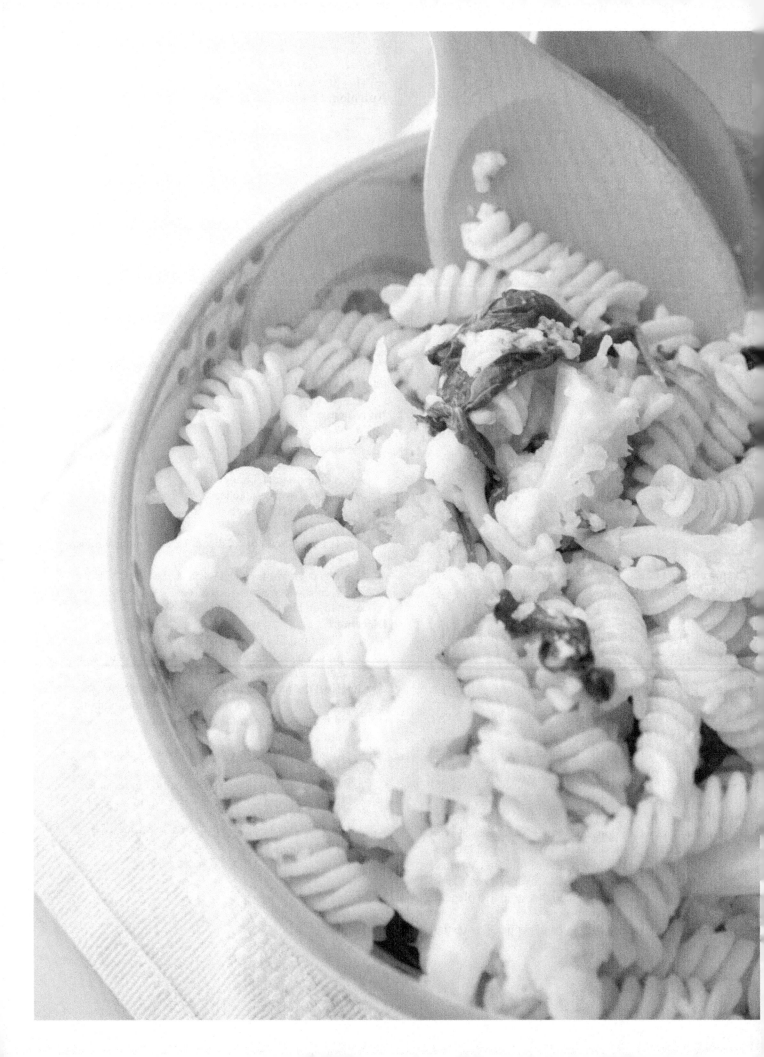

Chapter 9: Pasta and Noodles

85.   Vegetarian Pasta

Preparation Time: 5 minutes, **Cooking Time:** 16 minutes, **Difficulty Level:** Moderate, **Servings:** 4

Ingredients:
- 3 shallots, chopped
- ¼ tsp. red pepper flakes
- ¼ cup vegan parmesan cheese
- 2 Tbsp. olive oil
- 2 garlic cloves, minced
- 8 lb. spinach leaves
- 8 lb. linguine pasta
- 1 pinch salt
- 1 pinch black pepper

Directions:
1. In a large pot, boil water that is salted, then add pasta and cook for about 6 minutes. Drain the pasta in a colander.
2. Over medium heat, heat olive oil in a large skillet and add the shallots.
3. Cook for about 5 minutes until soft and caramelized, and stir in the spinach, garlic, red pepper flakes, salt, and black pepper.
4. Cook for about 5 minutes and add pasta and 2 ladles of pasta water.
5. Stir in the parmesan cheese and dish it out in a bowl to serve.

Nutrition: Calories: 284 kcal, Fat: 18.0 g, Protein: 29.0 g, Carbs: 1.5 g, Fiber: 0 g, Net Carbs: 1.5 g

86.   5-Ingredient Pasta

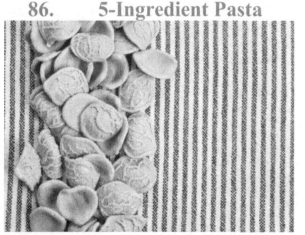

Preparation Time: 15 minutes, **Cooking Time:** 25 minutes, **Difficulty Level:** Moderate, **Servings:** 4

Ingredients:
- 1 (25 oz.) jar marinara sauce

- Olive oil, as needed
- 1 lb. dry vegan pasta
- 1 lb. assorted vegetables, like red onion, zucchini, and tomatoes
- ¼ cup prepared hummus
- Salt, to taste

Directions:
1. Preheat the oven to 400 °F. Grease a large baking sheet and arrange the vegetables in a single layer, then sprinkle with olive oil and salt.
2. Transfer into the oven and roast the vegetables for about 15 minutes.
3. In a large pot, boil water that is salted and cook the pasta according to the package directions.
4. Drain the water when the pasta is tender and put the pasta in a colander.
5. Mix the marinara sauce and hummus in a large pot to make a creamy sauce.
6. Stir in the cooked vegetables and pasta to the sauce and toss to coat well.
7. Dish out in a bowl and serve warm.

Nutrition: Calories: 415 kcal, Fat: 29.0 g, Protein: 33.0 g, Carbs: 5.5 g, Fiber: 2.0 g, Net Carbs: 3.5 g

87.   Asian Veggie Noodles

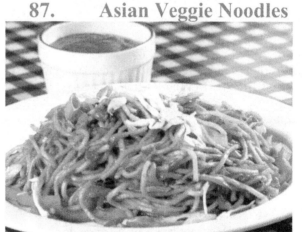

Preparation Time: 10 minutes, **Cooking Time:** 20 minutes, **Difficulty Level:** Easy, **Servings:** 4

Ingredients:
- ½ cup peas
- 1 tsp. rice vinegar
- 3 carrots, chopped
- 1 small packet of vermicelli
- 3 Tbsp. sesame oil
- 1 red pepper, chopped in small cubes
- 1 can baby corn
- 1 garlic clove, chopped

56

- 2 Tbsp. soy sauce
- 1 tsp. ginger powder
- ½ tsp. curry powder
- Salt and black pepper, to taste

Directions:
1. Take a bowl and add ginger powder, vinegar, soy sauce, curry powder, and a pinch of salt to it.
2. Add the noodles and cook them, following the instructions, then drain.
3. Heat the sesame oil and cook vegetables in it for 10 minutes on medium heat.
4. Add noodles to the mixture, then let it cook for 3 more minutes.
5. Remove from heat and serve to enjoy.

Nutrition: Calories: 329 kcal, Fat: 25.0 g, Protein: 20.0 g, Carbs: 6.0 g, Fiber: 1.0 g, Net Carbs: 5.0 g

88.   Asparagus Pasta

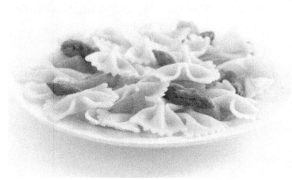

Preparation Time: 10 minutes, **Cooking Time:** 25 minutes, **Difficulty Level:** Moderate, **Servings:** 4

Ingredients:
- 8 oz. Farfalle Pasta, Uncooked
- 1 ½ Cups Asparagus, Fresh, Trimmed & Chopped into 1 Inch Pieces
- 1 Pint Grape Tomatoes, Halved
- 2 Tbsp.. Olive Oil
- Sea Salt & Black Pepper to Taste
- 2 Cups Mozzarella, Fresh & Drained
- ⅓ Cup Basil Leaves, Fresh & Torn
- 2 Tbsp.. Balsamic Vinegar

Directions:
1. First, heat the oven to 400 °F, then take out a stockpot. Cook your pasta per package instructions, and reserve ¼ cup of pasta water.
2. Get out a bowl, toss the tomatoes, oil, and asparagus, and season with salt and pepper. Spread this mixture on a baking sheet, as evenly as possible, and bake for fifteen minutes. Stir twice.

3. Remove your vegetables from the oven, and then add the cooked pasta to your baking sheet. Mix with a few tablespoons of pasta water so that your sauce becomes smoother.
4. Mix in your basil and mozzarella, drizzling with balsamic vinegar. Serve warm.

Nutrition: Calories: 920 kcal, Fats: 32 g, Carbs: 108 g, Proteins: 52 g

89.   Chickpea Pasta Salad

Preparation Time: 10 minutes, **Cooking Time:** 15 minutes, **Difficulty Level:** Moderate, **Servings:** 4

Ingredients:
- 2 Tbsp. Olive Oil
- 16 oz. Rotelle Pasta
- ½ Cup Cured Olives, Chopped
- 2 Tbsp. Oregano, Fresh & Minced
- 2 Tbsp. Parsley, Fresh & Chopped
- 1 Bunch Green Onions, Chopped
- ¼ Cup Red Wine Vinegar
- 15 oz. Canned Garbanzo Beans, Drained & Rinsed
- ½ Cup Parmesan Cheese, Grated
- Sea Salt and Black Pepper, to Taste

Directions:
1. Boil a pot of water and cook your pasta al dente per package instructions. Drain it and rinse it using cold water.
2. Get out a skillet and heat your olive oil over medium heat. Add in your scallions, chickpeas, parsley, oregano, and olives. Reduce the heat to low and cook for twenty minutes more. Allow this mixture to cool.
3. Toss your chickpea mixture with your pasta, and then add in your grated cheese, salt, pepper, and vinegar. Let pasta chill for four hours or overnight before serving.

Nutrition: Calories: 1235 kcal, Fats: 50 g, Carbs: 166 g, Proteins: 49 g

90.   Creamy Vegan Mushroom Pasta

Preparation Time: 10 minutes, **Cooking Time:** 30 minutes, **Difficulty Level:** Moderate, **Servings:** 4

Ingredients:
- 2 cups frozen peas, thawed
- 3 Tbsp. flour, unbleached
- 3 cups almond breeze, unsweetened
- 1 Tbsp. nutritional yeast

- ⅓ cup fresh parsley, chopped, plus extra for garnish
- ¼ cup olive oil
- 1 lb. pasta of choice
- 4 garlic cloves, minced
- ⅔ cup shallots, chopped
- 8 cups mixed mushrooms, sliced
- Salt and black pepper, to taste

Directions:
1. Take a bowl and boil pasta in salted water. In a pan over medium heat, warm up olive oil.
2. Add mushrooms, garlic, shallots, and ½ tsp. salt and cook for 15 minutes. Sprinkle flour on the vegetables and stir for a minute while cooking.
3. Add almond beverage, stir constantly. Let it simmer for 5 minutes, and add pepper to it.
4. Cook for 3 more minutes and remove from heat. Stir in nutritional yeast.
5. Add peas, salt, and pepper. Cook for another minute and add
6. Add pasta to this sauce. Garnish and serve!

Nutrition: Calories: 364 kcal, Fat: 28.0 g, Protein: 24.0 g, Carbs: 4.0 g, Fiber: 2.0 g, Net Carbs: 2.0 g

91. Creamy Vegan Pumpkin Pasta

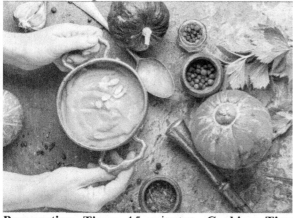

Preparation Time: 15 minutes, **Cooking Time:** 5 minutes, **Difficulty Level:** Moderate, **Servings:** 4

Ingredients:
- 12 oz. dried penne pasta
- 1 Tbsp. olive oil
- 1 cup raw cashews, soaked in water 4-8 hours, drained and rinsed
- 3 garlic cloves
- 1 cup pumpkin puree, canned
- 1 cup almond milk, plus more as needed
- ¼ tsp. ground nutmeg
- Fresh parsley, for garnish
- 1 Tbsp. lemon juice

- ¾ tsp. salt
- 1 Tbsp. fresh sage, chopped

Directions:
1. In a large pot, boil salted water. Add pasta and cook, following the package directions, and drain the pasta into a colander.
2. Dish out the pasta in a large serving bowl and add a dash of olive oil to prevent sticking.
3. Put the pumpkin, cashews, milk, lemon juice, garlic, salt, and nutmeg into the food processor and blend until smooth.
4. Stir in the sauce and sage over the pasta and toss to coat well.
5. Garnish with fresh parsley and dish out to serve hot.

Nutrition: Calories: 431 kcal, Fat: 31.0 g, Protein: 35.0 g, Carbs: 3.0 g, Fiber: 0.5 g, Net Carbs: 2.5 g

92. Creamy Vegan Spinach Pasta

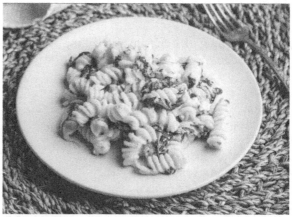

Preparation Time: 20 minutes, **Cooking Time:** 15 minutes, **Difficulty Level:** Moderate, **Servings:** 4

Ingredients:
- 2 Tbsp. lemon juice
- 1 cup raw cashews, for 8 hours soaked in water
- 1 Tbsp. olive oil
- 1½ cups vegetable broth
- 2 Tbsp. fresh dill, chopped
- Red pepper flakes, to taste
- 10 oz. dried fusilli
- ½ cup almond milk, unflavored and unsweetened
- 2 Tbsp. white miso paste
- 4 garlic cloves, divided
- 8 oz. fresh spinach, finely chopped
- ¼ cup scallions, chopped
- Salt and black pepper, to taste

Directions:
1. In a large pot, boil salted water and add pasta.

2. Cook according to the package directions and drain the pasta into a colander.
3. Dish out the pasta in a large serving bowl and add a dash of olive oil to prevent sticking.
4. Put the cashews, milk, miso, lemon juice, and 1 garlic clove into the food processor and blend until smooth.
5. Over medium heat, put olive oil in a large pot and add the remaining 3 garlic cloves.
6. Sauté for about 1 minute and stir in the spinach and broth.
7. Raise the heat and simmer for about 4 minutes until the spinach is bright green and wilted.
8. Stir in the pasta and cashew mixture and season with salt and black pepper.
9. Top with scallions and dill and dish out into plates to serve.

Nutrition: Calories: 94 kcal, Fat: 10.0 g, Protein: 0 g, Carbs: 1.0 g, Fiber: 0.3 g, Net Carbs: 0.7 g

93. Delicious Pasta Primavera

Preparation Time: 10 minutes, **Cooking Time:** 4 minutes, **Difficulty Level:** Moderate, **Servings:** 4

Ingredients:
- 8 oz. whole wheat penne pasta
- 1 Tbsp. fresh lemon juice
- 2 Tbsp. fresh parsley, chopped
- ¼ cup almonds slivered
- ¼ cup parmesan cheese, grated
- 14 oz. can tomato, diced
- ½ cup prunes
- ½ cup zucchini, chopped
- ½ cup asparagus, cut into 1-inch pieces
- ½ cup carrots, chopped
- ½ cup broccoli, chopped
- 1 ¾ cups vegetable stock
- Pepper
- Salt

Directions:
1. Add stock, tomatoes, parsley, prunes, zucchini, asparagus, carrots, and broccoli into the instant pot and stir well.
2. Seal pot with lid and cook on high for 4 minutes.
3. Once done, release pressure using quick release. Remove lid.
4. Add all of the remaining ingredients and stir well and serve.

Nutrition: Calories: 577 kcal, Fat: 57.3 g, Carbs: 19.7 g, Fiber: 6.1 g, Protein: 5.7 g

94. Flavorful Mac & Cheese

Preparation Time: 10 minutes, **Cooking Time:** 10 minutes, **Difficulty Level:** Moderate, **Servings:** 4

Ingredients:
- 16 oz. whole-grain elbow pasta
- 4 cups water
- 1 cup can tomato, diced
- 1 tsp. garlic, chopped
- 2 Tbsp. olive oil
- ¼ cup green onions, chopped
- ½ cup Parmesan cheese, grated
- ½ cup Mozzarella cheese, grated
- 1 cup Cheddar cheese, grated
- ¼ cup Passata
- 1 cup unsweetened almond milk
- 1 cup marinated artichoke, diced
- ½ cup sun-dried tomatoes, sliced
- ½ cup olives, sliced
- 1 tsp. salt

Directions:
1. Add pasta, garlic, water, tomatoes, oil, and salt into the instant pot and stir well.
2. With lid, seal the pot and cook on high for 4 minutes.
3. Once done, allow to release pressure naturally for 5 minutes, then release remaining using quick release. Remove the lid.
4. Set the pot on sauté mode. Add green onion, Parmesan cheese, Mozzarella cheese, Cheddar cheese, Passata, almond milk, artichoke, sun-dried tomatoes, and olive. Mix well.
5. Stir well and cook until the cheese is melted.
6. Serve and enjoy.

Nutrition: Calories: 577 kcal, Fat: 57.3 g, Carbs: 19.7 g, Fiber: 6.1 g, Protein: 5.7 g

95. Homemade Pasta Bolognese

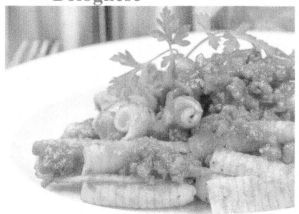

Preparation Time: 20 minutes, **Cooking Time:** 10 minutes, **Difficulty Level:** Moderate, **Servings:** 4

Ingredients:
- 17 oz. minced meat
- 12 oz. pasta
- 1piece sweet red onion
- 2 garlic cloves
- 1 Tbsp. vegetable oil
- 3 Tbsp. tomato paste
- 2 oz. grated parmesan cheese
- 3 pieces bacon

Directions:
1. Put finely chopped onions and garlic in a frying pan and fry in vegetable oil until you smell its aroma.
2. Add minced meat and chopped bacon to the pan. Constantly break the lumps with a spatula and mix so that the minced meat is crumbly.
3. Add tomato paste, grated Parmesan to the pan, mix, reduce heat, and leave to simmer when the mince is ready.
4. Currently, boil the pasta. I don't use saltwater because, for me, tomato paste and sauce as a whole turn out to be quite salty.
5. When the pasta is ready, discard it in a colander, arrange it on plates, add meat sauce with tomato paste on top of each serving.

Nutrition: Calories: 577 kcal, Fat: 57.3 g, Carbs: 19.7 g, Fiber: 6.1 g, Protein: 5.7 g

96. Loaded Creamy Vegan Pesto Pasta

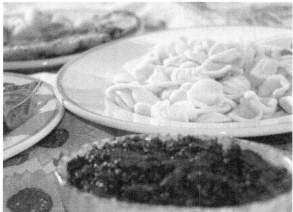

Preparation Time: 15 minutes, **Cooking Time:** 10 minutes, **Difficulty Level:** Moderate, **Servings:** 4

Ingredients:
- ¼ onion, finely chopped
- 8 romaine lettuce leaves
- 1 celery stalk, thinly sliced

- ½ cup blue cheese, crumbled
- 1 Tbsp. olive oil, plus a dash
- 1 cup almond milk, unflavored and unsweetened
- ½ cup vegan pesto
- 1 cup chickpeas, cooked
- 1 cup fresh arugula, packed
- 2 Tbsp. lemon juice
- Salt and black pepper, to taste
- 6 oz. orecchiette pasta, dried
- 1 cup full-fat coconut milk
- 2 Tbsp. whole wheat flour
- 1½ cups cherry tomatoes halved
- ½ cup Kalamata olives halved
- Red pepper flakes, to taste

Directions:
1. In a large pot, boil salted water. Add pasta and cook, following the package directions, and drain the pasta into a colander.
2. Dish out the pasta in a large serving bowl and add a dash of olive oil to prevent sticking.
3. Over medium heat, put olive oil in a large pot and whisk in the flour.
4. Cook for about 4 minutes until the mixture smells nutty, and stir in the coconut milk and almond milk.
5. For about 1 minute, let the sauce simmer and add the chickpeas, olives, and arugula.
6. Stir well and season with lemon juice, red pepper flakes, salt, and black pepper.
7. Dish out into plates and serve hot.

Nutrition: Calories: 220 kcal, Fat: 10.0 g, Protein: 31.0 g, Carbs: 1.5 g, Fiber: 0.5 g, Net Carbs: 1.0 g

97. Pasta with Garlic and Hot Pepper

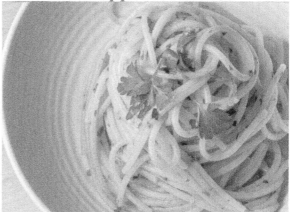

Preparation Time: 25 minutes, **Cooking Time:** 4 minutes, **Difficulty Level:** Easy, **Servings:** 4

Ingredients:
- 400g spaghetti

- 8 Tbsp.. extra-virgin olive oil
- 4 garlic cloves, chopped
- 1 chili pepper
- Coarse salt

Directions:
1. Boil water, add salt, and dip the spaghetti.
2. Meanwhile, in a saucepan, heat the oil with the garlic deprived of the inner and chopped germ and the chopped peppers. Be careful: the flame should be sweet, and the garlic should not darken.
3. Halfway through cooking, remove the spaghetti and continue cooking in the pan with the oil and garlic, adding the cooking water as if it were a risotto.
4. When cooked, serve the spaghetti.

Nutrition: Calories: 728 kcal, Fats: 20.92 g, Carbs: 108.16 g, Proteins: 20.16 g

98. Spaghetti in Spicy Tomato Sauce

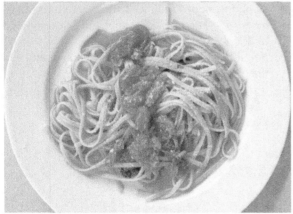

Preparation Time: 15 minutes, **Cooking Time:** 40 minutes, **Difficulty Level:** Hard, **Servings:** 4

Ingredients:
- 1-lb dried spaghetti
- 1 red bell pepper, diced
- 4 garlic cloves, minced
- 1 tsp. red pepper flakes, crushed
- 2 (14-oz.) cans of diced tomatoes
- 1 (6-oz.) can tomato paste
- 2 tsp. vegan sugar, granulated
- 2 Tbsp. olive oil
- 1 medium onion, diced
- 1 cup dry red wine
- 1 tsp. dried thyme
- ½ tsp. fennel seed, crushed
- 1½ cups coconut milk, full fat
- Salt and black pepper, to taste

Directions:
1. In a large pot, boil water. Add pasta, then cook according to the package directions and drain the pasta into a colander.
2. Dish out the pasta in a large serving bowl and add a dash of olive oil to prevent sticking.
3. Over medium heat, warm 2 tablespoons of olive oil and add garlic, onion, and bell pepper to a large pot.
4. Sauté for about 5 minutes and stir in the wine, thyme, fennel, and red pepper flakes.
5. Allow simmering on high heat for about 5 minutes until the liquid is reduced by about half.
6. Add diced tomatoes and tomato paste and allow to simmer for about 20 minutes, stirring occasionally.
7. Stir in the coconut milk and sugar and simmer for about 10 more minutes.
8. Season with salt and black pepper and pour the sauce over the pasta.
9. Toss to coat well and dish out in plates to serve.

Nutrition: Calories: 313 kcal, Fat: 25.0 g, Protein: 21.0 g, Carbs: 1.0 g, Fiber: 0 g, Net Carbs: 1.0 g

99. Spicy Sweet Chili Veggie Noodles

Preparation Time: 10 minutes, **Cooking Time:** 7 minutes, **Difficulty Level:** Moderate, **Servings:** 2

Ingredients:
- 1 head broccoli, cut into bite-sized florets
- 1 onion, finely sliced
- 1 Tbsp. olive oil
- 1 courgette, halved
- 2 nests whole-wheat noodles
- 150g mushrooms, sliced

For the Sauce:
- 3 Tbsp. soy sauce
- ¼ cup sweet chili sauce
- 1 tsp. Sriracha
- 1 Tbsp. peanut butter
- 2 Tbsp. boiled water

For the Topping:
- 2 tsp. sesame seeds
- 2 tsp. dried chili flakes

Directions:
1. On medium heat, warm up the olive oil, then add onions to a saucepan.
2. Sauté for about 2 minutes and add broccoli, courgette, and mushrooms.
3. Cook for about 5 minutes, stirring occasionally.
4. Whisk sweet chili sauce, soy sauce, Sriracha, water, and peanut butter in a bowl.

5. According to packet instructions, cook the noodles and add them to the vegetables.
6. Stir in the sauce and top with dried chili flakes and sesame seeds to serve.

Nutrition: Calories: 351 kcal, Fat: 27.0 g, Protein: 25.0 g, Carbs: 2.0 g, Fiber: 1.0 g, Net Carbs: 1.0 g

100. Stir Fry Noodles

Preparation Time: 10 minutes, **Cooking Time:** 10 minutes, **Difficulty Level:** Easy, **Servings:** 4

Ingredients:
- 1 cup broccoli, chopped
- 1 cup red bell pepper, chopped
- 1 cup mushrooms, chopped
- 1 large onion, chopped
- 1 batch Stir Fry Sauce, prepared
- Salt and black pepper, to taste
- 2 cups spaghetti, cooked
- 4 garlic cloves, minced
- 2 Tbsp. sesame oil

Directions:
1. In a pan over medium heat, heat sesame oil and add garlic, onions, bell pepper, broccoli, mushrooms.
2. Sauté for about 5 minutes and add spaghetti noodles and stir fry sauce.
3. Mix well and cook for 3 more minutes.
4. Dish out on plates and serve to enjoy.

Nutrition: Calories: 567 kcal, Fat: 48.0 g, Carbs: 6.0 g, Fiber: 4.0 g, Net Carbs: 2.0 g, Sodium: 373 mg, Protein: 33.0 g

101. Stuffed Pasta Shells

Preparation Time: 15 minutes, **Cooking Time:** 10 minutes, **Difficulty Level:** Moderate, **Servings:** 4

Ingredients:
- 5 cups Marinara Sauce
- 15 oz. Ricotta Cheese
- 1 ½ Cups Mozzarella Cheese, Grated
- ¾ Cup Parmesan Cheese, Grated
- 2 Tbsp.. Parsley, Fresh & Chopped
- ¼ Cup Basil Leaves, Fresh & Chopped
- 8 oz. Spinach, Fresh & Chopped
- ½ tsp.. Thyme
- Sea Salt & Black Pepper to Taste
- 1 lb. Ground Beef
- 1 Cup Onions, Chopped
- 4 Cloves Garlic, Diced
- 2 Tbsp.. Olive Oil, Divided
- 12 oz. Jumbo Pasta Shells

Directions:
1. Start by cooking your pasta shells by following your package instructions. Once they're cooked, then set them to the side.
2. Press sauté, and then add in half of your olive oil. Cook your garlic and onions, which should take about four minutes. Your onions should be tender, and your garlic should be fragrant.
3. Add your ground beef in, seasoning it with thyme, salt, and pepper, cooking for another four minutes.
4. Add in your basil, parsley, spinach, and marinara sauce.
5. Cover your pot and cook for five minutes on low pressure.
6. Use a quick release, and top with cheese.
7. Press sauté again, making sure that it stays warm until your cheese melts.
8. Take a Tbsp.. Of the mixture, stuffing it into your pasta shells.
9. Top with your remaining sauce before serving warm.

Nutrition: Calories: 1050 kcal, Fats: 51 g, Carbs: 90 g, Proteins: 57 g

102. Tuna Pasta

Preparation Time: 10 minutes, **Cooking Time:** 8 minutes, **Difficulty Level:** Moderate, **Servings:** 4

Ingredients:
- 10 oz. can tuna, drained
- 15 oz. whole wheat rotini pasta
- 4 oz. Mozzarella cheese, cubed
- ½ cup Parmesan cheese, grated
- 1 tsp. dried basil
- 14 oz. can tomato, diced
- 4 cups vegetable broth
- 1 Tbsp. garlic, minced
- 8 oz. mushrooms, sliced
- 2 zucchinis, sliced
- 1 onion, chopped
- 2 Tbsp.. olive oil
- Pepper and salt, to taste

Directions:
1. First, add oil into the inner pot of the instant pot and set the pot on sauté mode.
2. Add zucchini, mushrooms, and onion and sauté until onion is softened.
3. Add garlic and sauté for a minute.
4. Add basil, pasta, tuna, tomatoes, and broth and stir properly.
5. Shut the pot with a lid and cook on high for 4 minutes.

6. Once done, allow to naturally release pressure for 5 minutes, then release remaining using quick release. Remove the lid.
7. Add remaining ingredients. Stir properly and serve.

Nutrition: Calories: 361 kcal, Fats: 16 g, Carbs: 32 g, Proteins: 20 g

103. Vegan Bake Pasta with Bolognese Sauce and Cashew Cream

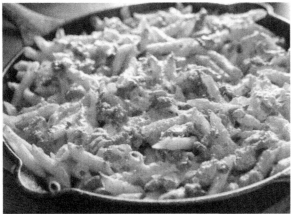

Preparation Time: 1 hour and 10 minutes, **Cooking Time:** 40 minutes, **Difficulty Level:** Hard
Servings: 4

Ingredients:
For the Pasta:
- 1 packet penne pasta

For the Bolognese Sauce:
- 1 Tbsp. soy sauce, 1 small can of lentils, 1 Tbsp. brown sugar, ½ cup tomato paste, 1 tsp. garlic, crushed, 1 Tbsp. olive oil, 2 tomatoes, chopped, 1 onion, chopped, 2 cups mushrooms, sliced
- Salt, Pepper, to taste

For the Cashew Cream:
- 1 cup raw cashews, ½ lemon, squeezed, ½ tsp. salt, ½ cup water

For the White Sauce:
- 1 tsp. black pepper, 1 tsp. Dijon mustard, ¼ cup nutritional yeast, Sea salt, as required, 2 cups coconut milk, 3 Tbsp. vegan butter, 2 Tbsp. all-purpose flour, ⅓ cup vegetable broth

Directions:
1. Take a pot and boil water, add pasta, boil for 3 minutes, and set aside. Fry onion and garlic, mushroom in olive oil, and add soy sauce to it.
2. Add sugar tomato paste, lentils, and canned tomato and let it simmer. Meanwhile, prepare the Bolognese sauce.

3. Season it with salt and black pepper. Add the lemon juice, cashews, water, and salt to the blender, blend for 2 minutes.
4. Add this to the sauce you have prepared and stir pasta in it. Melt the vegan butter in a saucepan, add in the flour, and stir.
5. Add vegetable stock and coconut milk to it and whisk well. Stir continuously and let it boil for about 5 minutes, then remove from heat.
6. Add Dijon mustard, nutritional yeast, black pepper, and sea salt. Preheat the oven to 430 °F.
7. Prepare a rectangular oven-safe dish by placing pasta and Bolognese sauce on it. Pour the white sauce on it and bake for a time of 20-25 minutes.

Nutrition: Calories: 314 kcal, Fat: 20.0 g, Protein: 31.0 g, Carbs: 2.5 g, Fiber: 0.8 g, Net Carbs: 1.7 g

104. Vegan Chinese Noodles

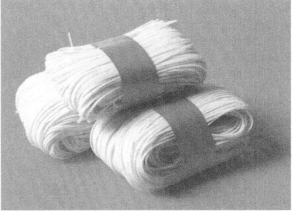

Preparation Time: 15 minutes, **Cooking Time:** 15 minutes, **Difficulty Level:** Moderate, **Servings:** 4

Ingredients:
- 300 g mixed oriental mushrooms, such as Oyster, Shiitake, and Enoki, cleaned and sliced
- 200 g thin rice noodles, cooked according to packet instructions and drained
- 2 garlic cloves, minced
- 1 fresh red chili
- 200 g courgettes, sliced
- 6 spring onions, reserving the green part
- 1 tsp. corn flour
- 1 Tbsp. agave syrup
- 1 tsp. sesame oil
- 100 g baby spinach, chopped
- Hot chili sauce, to serve
- 2(1-inch) pieces of ginger
- ½ bunch fresh coriander, chopped
- 4 Tbsp. vegetable oil
- 2 Tbsp. low-salt soy sauce
- ½ Tbsp. rice wine

- 2 limes to serve

Directions:
1. Over high heat in a large wok, heat sesame oil and add the mushrooms.
2. Sauté for about 4 minutes and add garlic, chili, ginger, courgette, coriander stalks, and the white part of the spring onions.
3. Sauté for about 3 minutes until softened and lightly golden.
4. Meanwhile, combine the corn flour and 2 tablespoons of water in a bowl.
5. Add soy sauce, agave syrup, sesame oil, and rice wine to the corn flour mixture.
6. Put this mixture in the pan to the veggie mixture and cook for about 3 minutes until thickened.
7. Add the spinach and noodles and mix well.
8. Stir in the coriander leaves and top with lime wedges, hot chili sauce, and reserved spring onions to serve.

Nutrition: Calories: 314 kcal, Fat: 22.0 g, Protein: 26.0 g, Carbs: 3.0 g, Fiber: 0.3 g, Net Carbs: 2.7 g

105.   Spaghetti Squash and Leeks

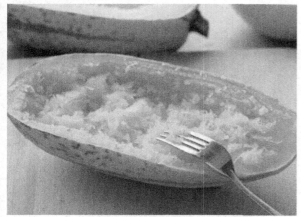

Preparation Time: 15 minutes, **Cooking Time:** 10 minutes, **Difficulty Level:** Moderate, **Servings:** 4

Ingredients:
- 2 leeks, sliced
- 1 tsp. chili powder
- 1 tsp. cumin, ground
- 1 tsp. onion powder
- 1 tsp. apple cider vinegar
- 1 lb. spaghetti squash, halved, seeds removed

- 1 Tbsp. Italian seasoning
- 1 cup water for cooking

Directions:
1. In the instant pot, pour water and insert the steamer rack.
2. Arrange spaghetti squash on the rack and close the lid.
3. Cook it on High for 10 minutes. Then allow natural pressure release for 5 minutes.
4. Check if the spaghetti squash is soft, shred the flesh with the help of a fork, and transfer to a bowl.
5. Add the rest of the ingred–ients, then toss and serve.

Nutrition: Calories: 110 kcal, Fat: 1.7 g, Fiber: 0 g, Carbs: 4.3 g, Protein: 0.8 g

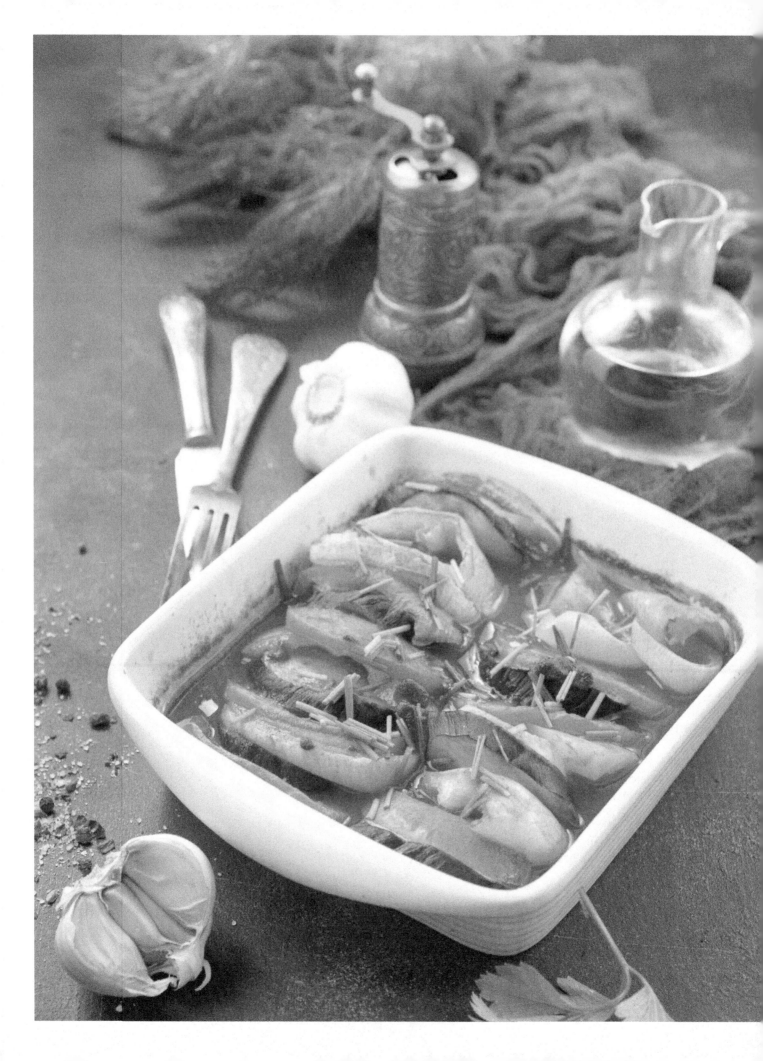

Chapter 10: Main

106. Cauliflower Salad

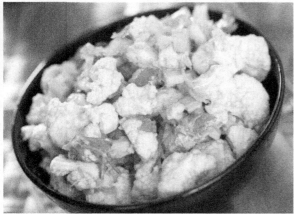

Preparation Time: 20 minutes, **Cooking Time:** 15 minutes, **Difficulty Level:** Moderate, **Servings:** 4

Ingredients:
- 8 cups cauliflower florets
- 5 Tbsp. olive oil, divided
- Salt and pepper, to taste
- 1 cup parsley
- 1 garlic clove, minced
- 2 Tbsp. lemon juice
- ¼ cup almonds, toasted and sliced
- 3 cups arugula
- 2 Tbsp. olives, sliced
- ¼ cup feta, crumbled

Directions:
1. Preheat your oven to 425 °F.
2. In a mixture of 1 tablespoon olive oil, salt, and pepper, toss the cauliflower.
3. Place the mixture into a baking pan. Roast this for 15 minutes.
4. Put the remaining oil, parsley, garlic, lemon juice, salt, and pepper in a blender.
5. Let this pulse until it becomes smooth.
6. In a salad bowl, place the roasted cauliflower.
7. Along with the parsley dressing, stir in the rest of the ingredients.

Nutrition: Calories: 198 kcal, Fat: 16.5 g, Saturated Fat: 3.0 g, Cholesterol: 6 mg, Sodium: 3 mg, Potassium: 570 mg, Carbohydrates: 10.4 g, Fiber: 4.1 g, Sugar: 4.0 g, Protein: 5.4 g

107. Cheesy Potato Casserole

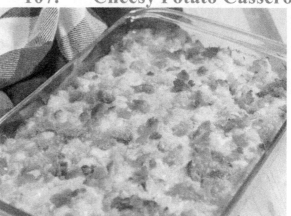

Preparation Time: 30 minutes, **Cooking Time:** 20 minutes, **Difficulty Level:** Moderate, **Servings:** 4

Ingredients:
- 1 white onion, finely chopped
- 2 oz. vegan butter
- ½ cup celery stalks, finely chopped
- Salt and black pepper, to taste
- 2 cups peeled and chopped potatoes
- 1 cup vegan mayonnaise
- 4 oz. freshly shredded vegan Parmesan cheese
- 1 green bell pepper, finely chopped and seeded
- 1 tsp. red chili flakes

Directions:
1. Preheat the oven to 400 °F. Spray a baking dish with cooking spray.
2. Season the celery, onion, and bell pepper with salt and black pepper.
3. In a bowl, mix the potatoes, vegan mayonnaise, Parmesan cheese, and red chili flakes.
4. Pour this new mixture into the baking dish, add the seasoned vegetables, and mix well.
5. Bake the mixture in the oven until golden brown, about 20 minutes.
6. Remove the baked potato and serve warm with baby spinach.

Nutrition: Calories: 577 kcal, Fat: 57.3 g, Carbs: 19.7 g, Fiber: 6.1 g, Protein: 9.3 g

108.   Coconut Brussels sprouts

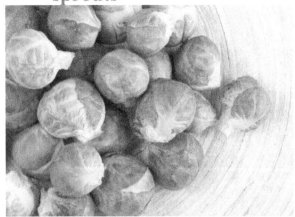

Preparation Time: 15 minutes, **Cooking Time:** 10 minutes, **Difficulty Level:** Easy, **Servings:** 4

Ingredients:
- 1 lb. Brussels sprouts, trimmed and sliced in half
- 1 Tbsp. soy sauce
- 2 Tbsp. coconut oil
- ¼ cup coconut water

Directions:
1. Add the coconut oil to a pan over medium heat. Cook the brussels sprouts for 4 minutes. Pour in the coconut water and cook for 3 minutes.
2. Add the soy sauce and cook for another 1 minute.

Nutrition: Calories: 114 kcal, Fat: 7.1 g, Saturated Fat: 5.7 g, Sodium: 269 mg, Potassium: 483 mg, Carbohydrates: 11.1 g, Fiber: 4.3 g, Sugar: 3.0 g, Protein: 4.0 g

109.   Rosemary Sweet Potato Medallions

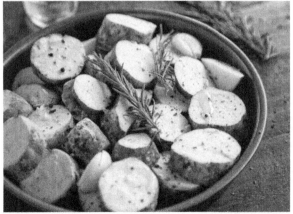

Preparation Time: 10 minutes, **Cooking Time:** 18 minutes, **Difficulty Level:** Moderate, **Servings:** 4

Ingredients:
- 4 sweet potatoes
- 2 Tbsp. coconut oil
- 1 cup water
- 1 Tbsp. rosemary
- 1 tsp. garlic powder
- Salt, to taste

Directions:
1. Add water and place the steamer rack over the water. Using a fork, prick sweet potatoes all over, then set on a steamer rack.
2. Shut the lid, cook for 12 minutes on High pressure, then release the pressure quickly and cut the sweet potatoes into ½ inch.
3. Melt the coconut oil on Sauté mode and add in the medallions.
4. Cook each side for 2 to 3 minutes until browned. Season with salt and garlic powder.
5. Add rosemary on top, then serve and enjoy!

Nutrition: Calories: 442 kcal, Fat: 19.5 g, Saturated Fat: 4.0 g, Carbohydrates: 41.3 g, Fiber: 8.0 g, Sugars: 22.2 g, Protein: 31.2 g

110.   Cod Stew with Rice & Sweet Potatoes

Preparation Time: 30 minutes, **Cooking Time:** 1 hour, **Difficulty Level:** Hard, **Servings:** 4

Ingredients:
- 2 cups water
- ¾ cup brown rice
- 1 Tbsp. vegetable oil
- 1 Tbsp. ginger, chopped
- 1 Tbsp. garlic, chopped
- 1 sweet potato, sliced into cubes
- 1 bell pepper, sliced
- 1 Tbsp. curry powder
- Salt to taste
- 15 oz. coconut milk
- 4 cod filets
- 2 tsp. freshly-squeezed lime juice
- 3 Tbsp. cilantro, chopped

Directions:
1. In a saucepan, place the water and rice. Bring the water and rice to a boil and simmer for 30 to 40 minutes then set aside.
2. Into a pan, pour the oil and heat over medium heat. Cook the garlic for 30 seconds.
3. Add the sweet potatoes and bell pepper. Season with curry powder and salt. Mix well.
4. Pour in the coconut milk. Simmer for 15 minutes.
5. Nestle the fish into the sauce and cook for another 10 minutes. Stir in the lime juice and cilantro.

6. Serve with the rice.

Nutrition: Calories: 382 kcal, Fat: 11.3 g, Saturated Fat: 4.8 g, Cholesterol: 45 mg, Sodium: 413 mg, Potassium: 736 mg, Carbohydrates: 49.5 g, Fiber: 5.3 g, Sugar: 8 g, Protein: 19.2 g

111. Curried Tofu with Buttery Cabbage

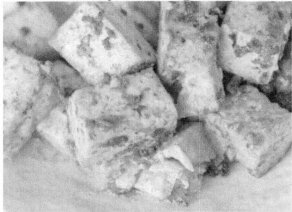

Preparation Time: 15 minutes, **Cooking Time:** 10 minutes, **Difficulty Level:** Easy, **Servings:** 4

Ingredients:
- 2 cups extra-firm tofu, pressed and cubed
- 1 Tbsp. + 3 ½ Tbsp. coconut oil
- ½ cup unsweetened shredded coconut
- 1 tsp. yellow curry powder
- 1 tsp. salt
- ½ tsp. onion powder
- 2 cups Napa cabbage
- 4 oz. vegan butter
- Salt and black pepper, to taste
- Lemon wedges for serving

Directions:
1. Add the tofu, 1 tablespoon of coconut oil, curry powder, salt, and onion powder in a medium bowl. Mix well until the tofu is well-coated with the spices.
2. In a non-stick skillet, heat the remaining coconut oil and fry the tofu until golden brown on all sides, 8 minutes. Divide onto serving plates and set aside for serving.
3. Melt half of the vegan butter in another skillet, and sauté the cabbage until slightly caramelized for 2 minutes. Season with salt, black pepper, and plate to the side of the tofu.
4. Melt the remaining vegan butter in the skillet and drizzle all over the cabbage.
5. Serve warm.

Nutrition: Calories: 432 kcal, Fat: 39 g, Carbohydrates: 9.94 g, Fiber: 4.6 g, Protein: 14.55 g

112. Curry Mushroom Pie

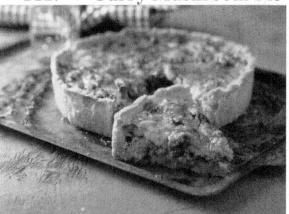

Preparation Time: 25 minutes, **Cooking Time:** 1 hour, **Difficulty Level:** Hard, **Servings:** 4

Ingredients:
For the Piecrust:
- 1 Tbsp. flax seed powder
- 3 Tbsp. water
- ¾ cup plain flour
- 4 Tbsp.. chia seeds
- 4 Tbsp. almond flour
- 1 Tbsp. nutritional yeast
- 1 tsp. baking powder
- 1 pinch salt
- 3 Tbsp. olive oil
- 4 Tbsp. water

For the Filling:
- 1 cup chopped baby Bella mushrooms
- 1 cup vegan mayonnaise
- 3 Tbsp. + 9 Tbsp. water
- ½ red bell pepper, finely chopped
- 1 tsp. curry powder
- ½ tsp. paprika powder
- ½ tsp. garlic powder
- ¼ tsp. black pepper
- ½ cup coconut cream
- 1¼ cups shredded vegan Parmesan cheese

Directions:
1. In two separate bowls, mix the different portions of flaxseed powder with the respective quantity of water. Allow soaking for 5 minutes.

For the Piecrust:
1. Preheat the oven to 350 °F.
2. When the flax egg is ready, pour the smaller quantity into a food processor and pour in all the ingredients for the pie crust. Blend until soft, smooth dough forms.

3. Line an 8-inch spring-form pan with parchment paper and grease with cooking spray.
4. In the bottom of the pan, spread the dough and bake for 15 minutes.

For the Filling:
1. In a bowl, add the remaining flax egg and all the filling's ingredients. Combine well and pour the mixture on the pie crust. Bake further for 40 minutes or until the pie is golden brown.
2. Remove from the oven and allow cooling for 1 minute.
3. Slice and serve the pie warm.

Nutrition: Calories: 577 kcal, Fat: 57.3 g, Carbs: 19.7 g, Fiber: 6.1 g, Protein: 5.7 g

113.   Garlic Mashed Potatoes & Turnips

Preparation Time: 20 minutes, **Cooking Time:** 30 minutes, **Difficulty Level:** Moderate, **Servings:** 4

Ingredients:
- 1 garlic head
- 1 tsp. olive oil
- 1 lb. turnips, sliced into cubes
- 2 lb. potatoes, sliced into cubes
- ½ cup almond milk
- ½ cup vegan parmesan cheese, grated
- 1 Tbsp. fresh thyme, chopped
- 1 Tbsp. fresh chives, chopped
- 2 Tbsp. vegan butter
- Salt and pepper to taste

Directions:
1. Preheat your oven to 375 °F.
2. Remove the extra papery peel from the garlic cloves without separating them. Remove the tip of the head, exposing the clove ends. Wrap the garlic in foil, spray with oil, then wrap in a package. Roast for 45 minutes, or until the garlic is golden brown and tender. So when cloves are cool enough to touch, squeeze them and any remaining oil off the foil into a small basin.
3. In a pot of water, boil the turnips and potatoes for 30 minutes or until tender.
4. Into a food processor, add all the ingredients along with the garlic.
5. Pulse until smooth.

Nutrition: Calories: 141 kcal, Fat: 3.2 g, Saturated Fat: 1.5 g, Cholesterol: 7 mg, Sodium: 284 mg, Potassium: 676 mg, Carbohydrates: 24.6 g, Fiber: 3.1 g, Sugar: 4.0 g, Protein: 4.6 g

114.   Green Beans with vegan Bacon

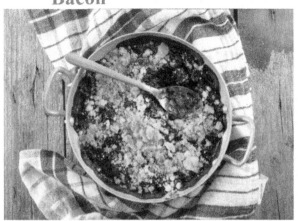

Preparation Time: 15 minutes, **Cooking Time:** 20 minutes, **Difficulty Level:** Easy, **Servings:** 4

Ingredients:
- 2 slices vegan bacon, chopped
- 1 shallot, chopped
- 24 oz. green beans
- Salt and pepper to taste
- ½ tsp. smoked paprika
- 1 tsp. lemon juice
- 2 tsp. vinegar

Directions:
1. Preheat your oven to 450 °F. Add the bacon to the baking pan and roast for 5 minutes.
2. Stir in the shallot and beans. Season with salt, pepper, and paprika.
3. Roast for 10 minutes.
4. Drizzle with lemon juice and vinegar.
5. Roast for another 2 minutes.

Nutrition: Calories: 49 kcal, Fat: 1.2 g, Saturated Fat: 0.4 g, Cholesterol: 3.0 mg, Sodium: 192 mg, Potassium: 249 mg, Carbohydrates: 8.1 g, Fiber: 3.0 g, Sugar: 4.0 g, Protein: 7.5 g

115.   Pecan & Blueberry Crumble

Preparation Time: 20 minutes, **Cooking Time:** 30 minutes, **Difficulty Level:** Moderate, **Servings:** 4

Ingredients:
- 14 oz. Blueberries
- 1 Tbsp. Lemon Juice, Fresh
- 1 ½ tsp. Stevia Powder
- 3 Tbsp. Chia Seeds
- 2 Cups Almond Flour, Blanched
- ¼ Cup Pecans, Chopped
- 5 Tbsp. coconut Oil

- 2 Tbsp. Cinnamon

Directions: Mix your blueberries, stevia, chia seeds, and lemon juice, and place it in an iron skillet.

1. Mix ingredients while spreading it over your blueberries.
2. Heat your oven to 400° F, and then transfer it to an oven-safe skillet, baking for a half hour.

Interesting Facts:

Blueberries are a delectable treat that is easily incorporated into many dishes. They are packed with antioxidants, and Vitamin C. Blueberries have been proven to promote eye health and slow macular degeneration.

Nutrition: Calories: 577 kcal, Fat: 57.3 g, Carbs: 19.7 g, Fiber: 6.1 g, Protein: 5.7 g

116.   Radish Chips

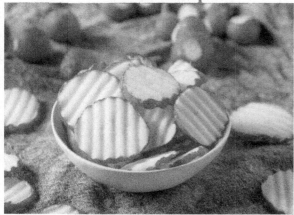

Preparation Time: 20 minutes, **Cooking Time:** 20 minutes, **Difficulty Level:** Moderate, **Servings:** 4

Ingredients:
- 10-15 radishes, Large
- Sea salt and black pepper, to taste

Directions:
1. Start by heating your oven to 375 °F.
2. Slice your radishes thin, and then spread them out on a cookie sheet that's been sprayed with cooking spray.
3. Mist the radishes with cooking spray, and then season with salt and pepper.
4. Bake for ten minutes, and then flip.
5. Bake for five to ten minutes more. They should be crispy.

Interesting Facts:

Potatoes are a great starchy source of potassium and protein. They are inexpensive if you are watching their budget. Bonus: Very heart healthy!

Nutrition: Calories: 577 kcal, Fat: 57.3 g, Carbs: 19.7 g, Fiber: 6.1 g, Protein: 5.7 g

117.   Roasted Sweet Potatoes

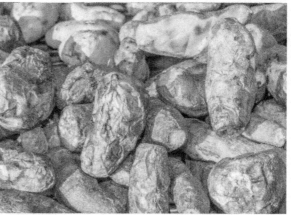

Preparation Time: 20 minutes, **Cooking Time:** 20 minutes, **Difficulty Level:** Moderate, **Servings:** 4

Ingredients:
- 2 potatoes, sliced into wedges
- 2 Tbsp. olive oil, divided
- Salt and pepper to taste
- 1 red bell pepper, chopped
- ¼ cup fresh cilantro, chopped
- 1 garlic, minced
- 2 Tbsp. almonds, toasted and sliced
- 1 Tbsp. lime juice

Directions:
1. Preheat your oven to 425 °F. In oil and salt, toss the sweet potatoes.
2. Transfer to a baking pan and roast the sweet potatoes for 20 minutes.
3. Combine the cilantro, red bell pepper, garlic, and almonds in a bowl.
4. Mix the remaining oil, lime juice, salt, and pepper in another bowl.
5. Combine this with the mixture of red bell pepper.
6. Serve sweet potatoes with a mixture of red bell pepper.

Nutrition: Calories: 146 kcal, Fat: 8.6 g, Saturated Fat: 1.1 g, Sodium: 317 mg, Potassium:380 mg, Carbohydrates:16 g,Fiber: 2.9 g, Sugar:5 g, Protein:12.5 g

118.   Smoked Tempeh with Broccoli Fritters

Preparation Time: 25 minutes, **Cooking Time:** 25 minutes, **Difficulty Level:** Moderate, **Servings:** 4

Ingredients:
For the Flax Egg:

- 4 Tbsp. flax seed powder
- 12 Tbsp. water

For the Grilled Tempeh:
- 3 Tbsp. olive oil
- 1 Tbsp. soy sauce
- 3 Tbsp. fresh lime juice
- 1 Tbsp. grated ginger
- Salt and cayenne pepper to taste
- 10 oz. tempeh slices

For the Broccoli Fritters:
- 2 cups rice broccoli
- 8 oz. tofu cheese
- 3 Tbsp. plain flour
- ½ tsp. onion powder
- 1 tsp. salt
- ¼ tsp. freshly ground black pepper
- 4¼ oz. vegan butter
- For serving:
- ½ cup mixed salad greens
- 1 cup vegan mayonnaise
- ½ lemon, juiced

Directions:
For the Smoked Tempeh:
1. In a bowl, mix the water with flaxseed powder and set it aside to soak for 5 minutes.
2. In another bowl, combine the olive oil, soy sauce, lime juice, grated ginger, salt, and cayenne pepper. Brush the tempeh slices with the mixture.
3. Over medium heat, heat a grill pan and grill the tempeh on both sides until nicely smoked and golden brown, 8 minutes. Transfer to a plate and set aside in a warmer for serving.
4. Combine the broccoli rice, tofu cheese, flour, onion, salt, and black pepper in a medium bowl. Mix in the flax egg until they are well combined and form 1-inch thick patties out of the mixture.
5. Melt the vegan butter in a medium skillet over medium heat and fry the patties on both sides until golden brown, 8 minutes. Remove the fritters onto a plate and set them aside.
6. In a small bowl, mix the vegan mayonnaise with the lemon juice.
7. Divide the smoked tempeh and broccoli fritters onto serving plates, add the salad greens, and serve vegan mayonnaise sauce.

Nutrition: Calories: 577 kcal, Fat: 57.3 g, Carbs: 19.7 g, Fiber: 6.1 g, Protein: 5.7 g

119.   Spicy Cheesy Tofu Balls

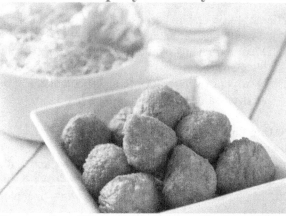

Preparation Time: 30 minutes, **Cooking Time:** 15 minutes, **Difficulty Level:** Moderate, **Servings:** 4

Ingredients:
- ⅓ cup vegan mayonnaise
- ¼ cup pickled jalapenos
- 1 pinch cayenne pepper
- 4 oz. grated vegan cheddar cheese
- 1 tsp. paprika powder
- 1 Tbsp. mustard powder
- 1 Tbsp. flax seed powder
- 3 Tbsp. water
- 2 ½ cup crumbled tofu
- Salt and black pepper to taste
- 2 Tbsp. vegan butter for frying

Directions:
For the Spicy Cheese:
1. Mix all the ingredients for the spicy vegan cheese in a bowl until well combined. Set aside.
2. In another medium bowl, combine the flax seed powder with water and allow soaking for 5 minutes.
3. Add the flax egg to the cheese mixture, the crumbled tofu, salt, and black pepper, and combine well. Use your hands to form large meatballs out of the mix.
4. Melt the vegan butter in a large skillet over medium heat and fry the tofu balls until they are cooked and golden brown on all sides, 10 minutes.
5. Serve the tofu balls with your favorite mashes or in burgers.

Nutrition: Calories: 371 kcal, Fat: 33.9 g, Carbs: 5.9 g, Fiber: 2.87 g, Protein: 14.5 g

120.   Tofu Cabbage Stir-Fry

Preparation Time: 15 minutes, **Cooking Time:** 10 minutes, **Difficulty Level:** Hard, **Servings:** 4

Ingredients:

- 5 oz. vegan butter
- 2 ½ cups baby, Bok choy, quartered lengthwise
- 8 oz sliced mushrooms
- 2 cups extra-firm tofu, pressed and cubed
- Salt and black pepper, to taste
- 1 tsp. onion powder
- 1 tsp. garlic powder
- 1 Tbsp. plain vinegar
- 2 garlic cloves, minced
- 1 tsp. chili flakes
- 1 Tbsp. fresh ginger, grated
- 3 scallions, sliced
- 1 Tbsp. sesame oil
- 1 cup vegan mayonnaise
- Wasabi paste, to taste
- Cooked white or brown rice (½ cup per person)

Directions:

1. Melt half of the vegan butter in a wok and sauté the Bok choy until softened, 3 minutes.
2. Season with salt, black pepper, onion powder, garlic powder, and vinegar. Sauté for 2 minutes to combine the flavors and plate the Bok choy.
3. Melt the remaining vegan butter in the wok and sauté the garlic, mushrooms, chili flakes, and ginger until fragrant.
4. Stir in the tofu and cook until browned on all sides. Add the scallions and Bok choy, heat for 2 minutes, and drizzle in the sesame oil.
5. Mix the vegan mayonnaise and wasabi in a small bowl, and mix into the tofu and vegetables. Cook for 2 minutes and dish the food.
6. Serve warm with steamed rice.

Nutrition: Calories: 522 kcal, Fat: 66.3 g, Carbs: 15.7 g, Fiber: 6.1 g, Protein: 16 g

121.   Simple Baked Okra

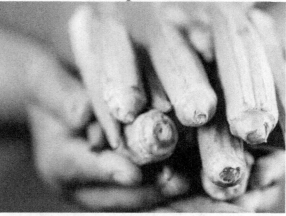

Preparation Time: 20 minutes, **Cooking Time:** 10 minutes, **Difficulty Level:** Moderate, **Servings:** 4

Ingredients:

- 8 oz. okra, chopped
- ½ tsp. ground black pepper
- ½ tsp. salt
- 1 Tbsp. olive oil

Directions:

1. Line the baking tray with foil. Place the okra in the tray in one layer.
2. Sprinkle the vegetables with ground black pepper and salt Mix up well. Then, drizzle the okra with olive oil.
3. Roast the vegetables in the preheated to 375 °F oven for 10 minutes.
4. Stir the okra with the help of a spatula every 3 minutes.

Nutrition: Calories: 49 kcal, Fat: 3.67 g, Carbs: 4.2 g, Fiber: 1.8 g, Protein: 1 g

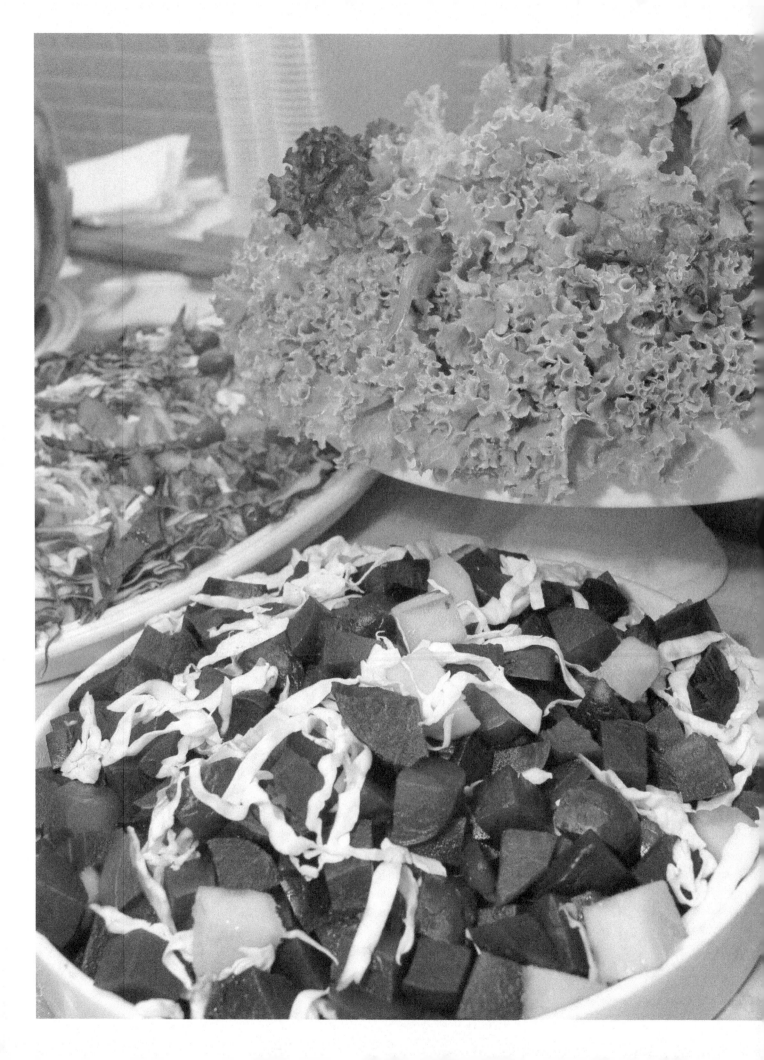

Chapter 11: Vegetable Salads

122.   Asparagus with Feta

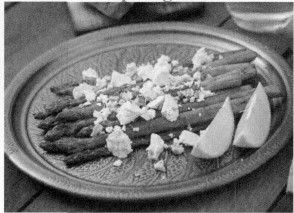

Preparation Time: 10 minutes, **Cooking Time:** 5 minutes, **Difficulty Level:** Easy, **Servings:** 4

Ingredients:
- 1 cup Feta cheese, cubed
- 1 lb. asparagus spears end trimmed
- 1 Tbsp. olive oil
- 1 cup of water
- 1 lemon
- Salt, to taste
- Freshly ground black pepper, to taste

Directions:
1. Add water into a pot and set trivet over the water.
2. Place steamer basket on the trivet.
3. Place the asparagus into the steamer basket.
4. Close the lid.
5. Cook for 1 minute on high pressure.
6. Release the pressure quickly.
7. Take a bowl and add olive oil to it.
8. Toss in asparagus until well-coated.
9. Season with pepper and salt.
10. Serve with feta cheese and lemon.
11. Enjoy!

Nutrition: Calories: 122 kcal, Fat: 9.34 g, Saturated Fat: 2.8 g, Cholesterol: 0 mg, Sodium: 439 mg, Carbohydrate: 5.5 g, Dietary Fiber: 2.2 g, Sugars: 3 g, Protein: 5.8 g, Vitamin D: 0 mcg, Calcium: 289 mg, Iron: 9 mg, Potassium: 1370 mg

123.   Buckwheat Salad

Preparation Time: 10 minutes, **Cooking Time:** 20 minutes, **Difficulty Level:** Moderate, **Servings:** 4

Ingredients:
- 1 cup raw buckwheat, rinsed

- 2 cups water
- 2 handful fresh baby spinach leaves, rinsed
- A handful of fresh basil leaves, rinsed
- 2 scallions, white parts only, rinsed and chopped
- 1 lemon zest
- ½ lemon juice
- ½ red onion, finely chopped
- Himalayan pink salt, to taste
- Freshly ground black pepper, to taste
- ¼ cup extra-virgin olive oil
- 1 red chili, rinsed and thinly sliced
- 2 Tbsp. mixed sprouts, rinsed
- 1 ripe avocado, peeled, pitted, and sliced
- 1½ oz. Feta cheese (optional)

Directions:
1. Mix the buckwheat and water, then bring it to a boil over high heat. Reduce the heat to simmer and cook for 15 minutes, or until soft. Remove from the heat and let cool.
2. Meanwhile, combine the baby spinach, basil, scallions, lemon zest, and lemon juice in a food processor and process for 30 seconds. Stir the herb mixture into the cooled buckwheat.
3. Add the red onion and season with salt and pepper. Arrange the buckwheat on a platter. Drizzle with the olive oil and scatter on the chopped chili and sprouts. Top with the sliced avocado, crumble the feta over the top (if using), and serve.

Nutrition: Calories: 350 kcal, Fat: 28.0 g, Fiber: 1.0 g, Carbs: 8.0 g, Protein: 22.0 g

124.   Chickpea and Spinach Salad

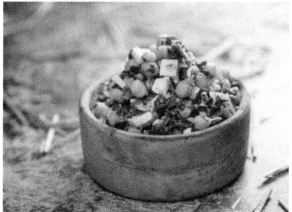

Preparation Time: 5 minutes, **Cooking Time:** 0 minutes, **Difficulty Level:** Easy, **Servings:** 4

Ingredients:
- 2 cans (14.5 oz. each) chickpeas, drained andrinsed
- 7 oz. vegan feta cheese, crumbled or chopped
- 1 Tbsp. lemon juice
- ⅓ -½ cup olive oil
- ½ tsp. salt or to taste
- 4-6 cups spinach, torn
- ½ cup raisins
- 2 Tbsp. honey
- 1-2 tsp. ground cumin
- 1 tsp. chili flakes

Directions:
1. Add cheese, chickpeas, and spinach into a large bowl.
2. Add the rest of the ingredients into another bowl to make the dressing and mix well.
3. Pour dressing over the salad. Toss well and serve.

Nutrition: Calories: 607 kcal, Fat: 37.18 g, Saturated Fat: 15.7 g, Cholesterol: 0 mg, Sodium: 974 mg, Carbohydrate: 60 g, Dietary Fiber: 9.8 g, Sugars: 25 g, Protein: 11 g, Vitamin D: 0 mcg, Calcium: 104 mg, Iron: 3 mg, Potassium: 498 mg

125. Colorful Protein Power Salad

Preparation Time: 20 minutes, **Cooking Time:** 15 minutes, **Difficulty Level:** Moderate, **Servings:** 4

Ingredients:
- ½ cup dry quinoa
- 2 cups dry navy beans
- 1 green onion, chopped
- 2 tsp.. garlic, minced
- 3 cups green or purple cabbage, chopped
- 4 cups kale, fresh or frozen, chopped
- 1 cup shredded carrot, chopped
- 2 Tbsp.. extra virgin olive oil
- 1 tsp.. lemon juice
- ¼ tsp. Salt
- ¼ tsp. pepper

Directions:
1. Prepare the quinoa according to the recipe.
2. Prepare the beans according to the method.
3. In a frying pan, heat a tablespoon of olive oil over medium heat.
4. Add the chopped green onion, garlic, and cabbage, and sauté for 2-3 minutes.
5. Add the kale, the remaining 1 tablespoon of olive oil, and salt. Lower the heat and cover until the greens have wilted (around 5 minutes). Take the pan from the stove and set it aside.

6. Take a large bowl and mix the remaining ingredients with the kale and cabbage mixture once it has cooled down. Add more salt and pepper to taste.
7. Mix until everything is distributed evenly.
8. Serve topped with a dressing, or store for later!

Nutrition: Calories: 1100 kcal, Fat: 19.9 g, Saturated Fat: 2.7 g, Cholesterol: 0 mg, Sodium: 420 mg, Carbohydrate: 180.8 g, Dietary Fiber: 60.1 g, Sugars: 14.4 g, Protein: 58.6 g, Vitamin D: 0 mcg, Calcium: 578 mg, Iron: 16 mg, Potassium: 3755 mg,

126. Vegetable Medley

Preparation Time: 10 minutes, **Cooking Time:** 3 minutes, **Difficulty Level:** Easy, **Servings:** 4

Ingredients:
- 2 carrots, peeled and cut on the bias
- 16 asparagus, trimmed
- 1 small head cauliflower, broken into florets
- 1 small head broccoli, broken into florets
- 5 oz. green beans
- 1 cup of water
- Salt to taste

Directions:
1. Add water and set the trivet on top of the water. Place steamer basket on top.
2. Spread green beans, cauliflower, asparagus, carrots, broccoli in a steamer basket. Close the lid.
3. Steam for 3 minutes on High. Release the pressure quickly.
4. Season with salt, serve, and enjoy!

Nutrition: Carbs: 24.7 g kcal, Protein: 9.5 g, Fats: 10.8 g, Calories: 248

127. Edamame & Ginger Citrus Salad

Preparation Time: 15 minutes, **Cooking Time:** 0 minutes, **Difficulty Level:** Easy, **Servings:** 4

Ingredients:
For the Dressing:
- ¼ cup orange juice
- 1 tsp. lime juice
- ½ Tbsp. maple syrup
- ½ tsp. ginger, finely minced
- ½ Tbsp.. sesame oil
For the Salad:
- ½ cup dry green lentils
- 2 cups carrots, shredded
- 4 cups kale, fresh or frozen, chopped

- 1 cup edamame, shelled
- 1 Tbsp. roasted sesame seeds
- 2 tsp. mint, chopped
- Salt and pepper to taste
- 1 small avocado, peeled, pitted, diced

Directions:
1. Prepare the lentils according to the method.
2. Combine the orange and lime juices, maple syrup, and ginger in a small bowl. Mix with a whisk while slowly adding the sesame oil.
3. Add the cooked lentils, carrots, kale, edamame, sesame seeds, and mint to a large bowl.
4. Add the dressing and stir well until all the ingredients are coated evenly.
5. Store or serve topped with avocado and an additional sprinkle of mint.

Nutrition: Calories: 507 kcal, Fat: 23.1 g, Saturated Fat: 4.0 g, Cholesterol: 0 mg, Sodium: 303 mg, Carbohydrate: 56.8 g, Dietary Fiber: 21.6 g, Sugars: 8.4 g, Protein: 24.6 g, Vitamin D: 0 mcg, Calcium: 374 mg, Iron: 8 mg, Potassium: 1911 mg

128.   Greek Style Beans

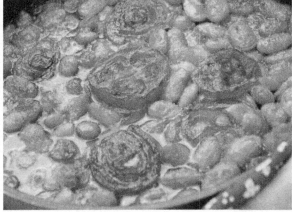

Preparation Time: 10 minutes, **Cooking Time:** 10 hours and 40 minutes, **Difficulty Level:** Hard, **Servings:** 4

Ingredients:
- 3 cups white beans
- ¼ cup olive oil
- 1 onion, diced
- 1 garlic, clove peeled
- 28 oz. canned crushed tomatoes

Directions:
1. Into the Instant Pot, pour 8 cups of water. Then add the white beans. Season with a pinch of salt. Let the beans soak for up to 10 hours.
2. Seal the pot. Set it to manual. Choose bean/chili function. Set the Timer to about 15 minutes at high pressure. Release the pressure naturally.

3. Transfer the white beans into a bowl and set them aside. Set aside 1 cup of the cooking liquid.
4. Drain the remaining liquid. Press the sauté setting. Heat the olive oil. Cook the onion, garlic, and tomatoes for 5 minutes.
5. Add the reserved cooking liquid and the tomatoes. Put the beans back. Stir well. Secure the pot.
6. Choose bean/chili function for 5 minutes at high pressure. Release the pressure naturally.
7. Season with salt and pepper.

Nutrition: Carbs: 24.7 g, Protein: 9.5 g, Fats: 10.8 g, Calories: 248 kcal

129.   Herby-Garlic Potatoes

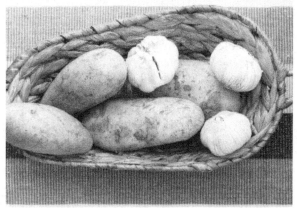

Preparation Time: 10 minutes, **Cooking Time:** 15 minutes, **Difficulty Level:** Moderate, **Servings:** 4

Ingredients:
- 1½ lb. potatoes
- 3 Tbsp. coconut oil
- ½ cup vegetable broth
- 2 Tbsp. fresh rosemary, chopped
- 3 garlic cloves, thinly chopped
- ½ tsp. fresh thyme, chopped
- ½ tsp. fresh parsley, chopped
- ¼ tsp. black pepper, ground

Directions:
1. Take a small knife and pierce each potato to ensure there are no blowouts. Then place under pressure.
2. Melt coconut oil on Sauté mode. Add potatoes, rosemary, thyme, garlic, parsley, and pepper and cook for 10 minutes.
3. Take a bowl, mix miso paste and vegetable stock, and stir in the mixture in the instant pot.
4. Shut the lid and cook for 5 minutes on High pressure and release the pressure quickly.
5. Serve with parsley on top and enjoy!

Nutrition: Carbs: 33.3 g, Protein: 14.6 g, Fats: 26.6 g, Calories: 456 kcal

130.   Grilled Veggie and Hummus Wrap

Preparation Time: 15 minutes, **Cooking Time:** 10 minutes, **Difficulty Level:** Moderate, **Servings:** 4

Ingredients:
- 1 large eggplant
- 1 large onion
- ½ cup extra-virgin olive oil
- 6 lavash wraps or large pita bread
- 1 cup creamy traditional hummus

Directions:
1. Preheat a grill, large grill pan, or lightly oiled large skillet on medium heat.
2. Slice the eggplant and onion into circles. Rub the vegetables with olive oil and sprinkle with salt.
3. Cook the vegetables on both sides, about 3 to 4 minutes on each side.
4. To make the wrap, lay the lavash or pita flat. Scoop 3 tablespoons of hummus on the wrap.
5. Evenly divide the vegetables among the wraps, layering them along one side of the wrap. Gently fold over the side of the wrap with the vegetables, tucking them in and making a tight wrap.
6. Lay the wrap seam-side-down and cut in half or thirds.
7. You can also wrap each sandwich with plastic wrap to help it hold its shape and eat it later.

Nutrition: Carbs: 24.7 g, Protein: 9.5 g, Fats: 10.8 g, Calories: 248 kcal

131.   Lebanese Potato Salad

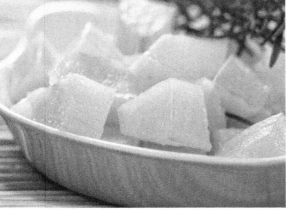

Preparation Time: 5 minutes, **Cooking Time:** 10 minutes, **Difficulty Level:** Moderate, **Servings:** 4

Ingredients:
- 1lb. Russet potatoes
- 1 ½ Tbsp. extra virgin olive oil
- 2 scallions, thinly sliced
- Freshly ground pepper to taste
- 2 Tbsp. lemon juice
- ¼ tsp. salt or to taste
- 2 Tbsp. fresh mint leaves, chopped

Directions:
1. Place a saucepan half-filled with water over medium heat. Add salt and potatoes and cook for 10 minutes until tender. Drain the potatoes. Place the potatoes in a bowl of cold water to cool them down. When cool enough to handle, peel and cube the potatoes. Place in a bowl.

To Make the Dressing:
1. Add oil, lemon juice, salt, and pepper in a bowl and whisk well. Drizzle dressing over the potatoes. Toss well.
2. Add scallions and mint and toss well.
3. Divide into 4 plates and serve.

Nutrition: Calories: 129 kcal, Fat: 5.5 g, Saturated Fat: 0.9 g, Cholesterol: 0 mg, Sodium: 158 mg, Carbohydrate: 18.8 g, Dietary Fiber: 3.2 g, Sugars: 1.6 g, Protein: 2.2 g, Vitamin D: 0 mcg, Calcium: 22 mg, Iron: 1 mg, Potassium: 505 mg

132.   Lentil Radish Salad

Preparation Time: 15 minutes, **Cooking Time:** 0 minutes, **Difficulty Level:** Easy, **Servings:** 4

Ingredients:
For the Dressing:
- 1 Tbsp.. extra virgin olive oil
- 1 Tbsp.. lemon juice
- 1 Tbsp.. maple syrup
- 1 Tbsp.. water
- ½ Tbsp.. sesame oil
- 1 Tbsp.. Miso paste, yellow or white
- ¼ tsp.. salt
- ¼ tsp. pepper

For the Salad:
- ½ cup dry chickpeas
- ¼ cup dry green or brown lentils
- 1 14-oz. pack of silken tofu
- 5 cups mixed greens, fresh or frozen
- 2 radishes, thinly sliced
- ½ cup cherry tomatoes halved
- ¼ cup roasted sesame seeds

Directions:
1. Prepare the chickpeas according to the method. Prepare the lentils according to the method.
2. In a blender or food processor, put all the ingredients for the dressing. Mix on low until

smooth while adding water until it reaches the desired consistency.

3. Add salt, pepper (to taste), and optionally more water to the dressing; set aside. Cut the tofu into bite-sized cubes.

4. Combine the mixed greens, tofu, lentils, chickpeas, radishes, and tomatoes in a large bowl. Add the dressing and mix everything until it is coated evenly.

5. Top with the optional roasted sesame seeds, if desired. Refrigerate before serving and enjoy, or store for later!

Nutrition: Calories: 621 kcal, Fat: 19.6 g, Saturated Fat: 2.8 g, Cholesterol: 0 mg, Sodium: 996 mg, Carbohydrate: 82.7 g, Dietary Fiber: 26.1 g, Sugars: 20.7 g, Protein: 31.3 g, Vitamin D: 0 mcg, Calcium: 289 mg, Iron: 9 mg, Potassium: 1370 mg

133.   Mashed Potatoes with Spinach

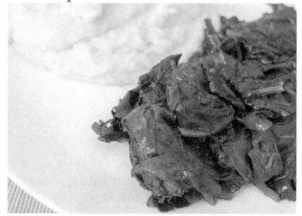

Preparation Time: 10 minutes, **Cooking Time:** 10 minutes, **Difficulty Level:** Moderate, **Servings:** 4

Ingredients:
- 2 cups spinach, chopped
- 3 lb. potatoes, peeled and quartered
- ½ cup almond milk
- ⅓ cup coconut oil
- 2 Tbsp. fresh chives, chopped
- 1½ cups of water
- Salt and black pepper, to taste

Directions:
1. Add water, salt, and potatoes to your cooker. Close the lid.
2. Cook for 8 minutes on High pressure. Release the pressure quickly.
3. Take a bowl, drain the potatoes, and reserve the liquid in the bowl.
4. Take another bowl and mash the potatoes. Mix with coconut oil and almond milk.

5. Season with salt and pepper, then add the reserved cooking liquid and thin the potatoes to attain the desired consistency.

6. Put the spinach in the remaining potato liquid and keep stirring. Season it.

7. Drain and serve with potato mash, and then garnish with chives and black pepper.

8. Serve and enjoy!

Nutrition: Calories: 442 kcal, Fat: 19.5 g, Saturated Fat: 4.0 g, Carbohydrates: 41.3 g, Fiber: 8 g, Sugars: 22.2 g, Protein: 31.2 g

134.   Roasted Almond Protein Salad

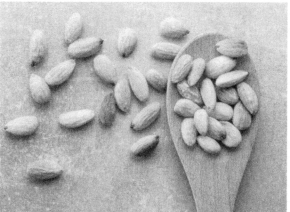

Preparation Time: 30 minutes, **Cooking Time:** 15 minutes, **Difficulty Level:** Moderate, **Servings:** 4

Ingredients:
- ½ cup dry quinoa
- ½ cup dry navy beans
- ½ cup dry chickpeas
- ½ cup raw whole almonds
- 1 tsp. extra virgin olive oil
- ½ tsp. salt
- ½ tsp. paprika
- ½ tsp. cayenne
- Dash chili powder
- 4 cups spinach, fresh or frozen
- ¼ cup purple onion, chopped

Directions:
1. Prepare the quinoa according to the recipe. Store in the fridge for now.
2. Prepare the beans according to the method. Store in the fridge for now.
3. Toss the almonds, olive oil, salt, and spices in a large bowl, and stir until the ingredients are evenly coated.
4. Put a skillet over medium-high heat, and transfer the almond mixture to the heated skillet.

5. Roast while stirring until the almonds are browned, around 5 minutes. You may hear the ingredients pop and crackle in the pan as they warm up. Stir frequently to prevent burning.
6. Shut the heat and toss the cooked and chilled quinoa and beans, onions, and spinach or mixed greens in the skillet. Stir well before transferring the roasted almond salad to a bowl.
7. Enjoy the salad with a dressing of choice, or store for later!

Nutrition: Calories: 347 kcal, Fat: 10.5 g, Saturated Fat: 1.0 g, Cholesterol: 0 mg, Sodium: 324 mg, Carbohydrate: 49.2 g, Dietary Fiber: 14.7 g, Sugars: 4.7 g, Protein: 17.2 g, Vitamin D: 0 mcg, Calcium: 139 mg, Iron: 5 mg, Potassium: 924 mg

135.   Shaved Brussel Sprout Salad

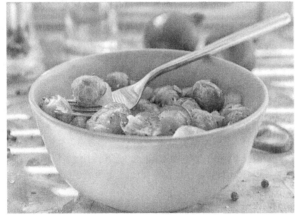

Preparation Time: 25 minutes, **Cooking Time:** 0 minutes, **Difficulty Level:** Easy, **Servings:** 4

Ingredients:
For the Dressing:
- 1 Tbsp. brown mustard
- 1 Tbsp. maple syrup
- 2 Tbsp. apple cider vinegar
- 2 Tbsp. Extra virgin olive oil
- ½ Tbsp. garlic minced

For the Salad:
- ½ cup dry red kidney beans
- ¼ cup dry chickpeas
- 2 cups Brussel sprouts
- 1 cup purple onion
- 1 small sour apple
- ½ cup slivered almonds, crushed
- ½ cup walnuts, crushed
- ½ cup cranberries, dried
- ¼ tsp. Salt
- ¼ tsp. pepper

Directions:

1. Prepare the beans according to the method. Mix the dressing ingredients in a bowl and stir properly until combined.
2. Refrigerate the dressing for up to one hour before serving. Use a grater, mandolin, or knife to slice each Brussel sprout thinly. Repeat this with the apple and onion.
3. Take a large bowl to mix the chickpeas, beans, sprouts, apples, onions, cranberries, and nuts. Drizzle the cold dressing over the salad to coat.
4. Serve with salt and pepper to taste, or store for later!

Nutrition: Calories: 432 kcal, Fat: 23.5 g, Saturated Fat: 2.2 g, Cholesterol: 0 mg, Sodium: 197 mg, Carbohydrate: 45.3 g, Dietary Fiber: 12.4 g, Sugars: 14 g, Protein: 15.9 g, Vitamin D: 0 mcg, Calcium: 104 mg, Iron: 4 mg, Potassium: 908 mg

136.   Southwest Style Salad

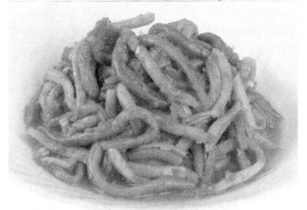

Preparation Time: 10 minutes, **Cooking Time:** 0 minutes, **Difficulty Level:** Easy, **Servings:** 4

Ingredients:
- ½ cup dry black beans
- ½ cup dry chickpeas
- ⅓ cup purple onion, diced
- 1 red bell pepper, pitted, sliced
- 4 cups mixed greens, fresh or frozen, chopped
- 1 cup cherry tomatoes, halved or quartered
- 1 medium avocado, peeled, pitted, and cubed
- 1 cup sweet kernel corn, canned, drained
- ½ tsp.. chili powder
- ¼ tsp.. cumin
- ¼ tsp. Salt
- ¼ tsp. pepper
- 2 tsp.. olive oil
- 1 Tbsp.. vinegar

Directions:
1. Prepare the black beans and chickpeas according to the method.
2. Put all the ingredients into a large bowl.

3. Toss the mix of veggies and spices until combined thoroughly.
4. Store, or serve chilled with some olive oil and vinegar on top.

Nutrition: Calories: 635 kcal, Fat: 19.9 g, Saturated Fat: 3.6 g, Cholesterol: 0 mg, Sodium: 302 mg, Carbohydrate: 95.4 g, Dietary Fiber: 28.1 g, Sugars: 18.8 g, Protein: 24.3 g, Vitamin D: 0 mcg, Calcium: 160 mg, Iron: 7 mg, Potassium: 1759mg

137.   Spanish Green Beans

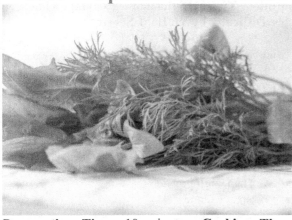

Preparation Time: 10 minutes, **Cooking Time:** 20 minutes, **Difficulty Level:** Easy, **Servings:** 4

Ingredients:
- 1 large onion, chopped
- 4 garlic cloves, finely chopped
- 1- lb. green beans, fresh or frozen, trimmed
- 1 (15-oz.) can diced tomatoes

Directions:
1. In a huge pot over medium heat, cook olive oil, onion, and garlic; cook for 1 minute.
2. Cut the green beans into 2-inch pieces.
3. Add the green beans and 1 tsp. of salt to the pot and toss everything together; cook for 3 minutes.
4. Add the diced tomatoes, remaining ½ tsp. of salt, and black pepper to the pot; continue to cook for another 12 minutes, stirring ccasionally.
5. Serve warm.

Nutrition: Calories: 577 kcal, Fat: 57.3 g, Carbs: 19.7 g, Fiber: 6.1 g, Protein: 5.7 g

138.   Spinach & Dill Pasta Salad

Preparation Time: 10 minutes, **Cooking Time:** 45 minutes, **Difficulty Level:** Moderate, **Servings:** 4

Ingredients:
- 1lb. potatoes, peeled and cut into bite-sized pieces
- 2 Tbsp. coconut oil, unsalted
- 3 Tbsp. olive oil
- 2 cups vegetable broth
- 2 carrots, peeled and chopped
- 3 celery stalks, chopped
- 2 onions, peeled and chopped
- 1 zucchini, cut into ½ inch thick slices
- 1 Tbsp. paprika
- 1 Tbsp. salt
- 1 tsp. black pepper
- A handful of fresh celery leaves

Directions:
1. Warm oil on Sauté mode. Stir-fry onions for 3-4 minutes.
2. Add celery, zucchini, carrots, and ¼ cup broth. Cook for 10 minutes more and keep stirring continuously. Stir in potatoes, cayenne pepper, bay leaves, remaining broth, celery, salt, and pepper.
3. Close the lid. Cook at Meat/Stew for 30 minutes on High. Quick-release the pressure.
4. Serve and enjoy!

Nutrition: Carbs: 24. 7 g, Protein: 19.5 g, Fats: 10.8 g, Calories: 248 kcal

139.   Steamed Artichoke with Lemon Aioli

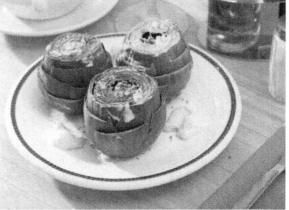

Preparation Time: 10 minutes, **Cooking Time:** 10 minutes, **Difficulty Level:** Moderate, **Servings:** 4

Ingredients:
- 4 artichokes, trimmed
- 1 lemon, halved
- 1 tsp. lemon zest
- 1 Tbsp. lemon juice
- 3 cloves garlic, crushed
- ½ cup mayonnaise

- 1 cup of water
- 1 handful parsley, chopped
- Salt, to taste

Directions:
1. Cut the artichoke's ends, rub with lemon. Add water into the pot.
2. Set steamer basket on top. Add artichoke into your basket and point this upward. Then sprinkle some salt.
3. Shut the lid, cook for 10 minutes on High pressure, then release the pressure quickly. Take a mixing bowl, add lemon juice, garlic, mayonnaise, and lemon zest.
4. Season with salt and serve with parsley on top and enjoy!

Nutrition: Calories: 256 kcal, Fat: 21.4 g, Carbs: 8.79 g, Fiber: 3.8 g, Protein: 2.43 g

140.   Super Summer Salad

Preparation Time: 10 minutes, **Cooking Time:** 0 minutes, **Difficulty Level:** Moderate, **Servings:** 4

Ingredients:
For the Dressing:
- 1 Tbsp.. olive oil
- ¼ cup chopped basil
- 1 tsp.. lemon juice
- ¼ tsp. Salt
- 1 medium avocado, halved, diced
- ¼ cup water

For the Salad:
- ¼ cup dry chickpeas
- ¼ cup dry red kidney beans
- 4 cups raw kale, shredded
- 2 cups Brussel sprouts, shredded
- 2 radishes, thinly sliced
- 1 Tbsp.. walnuts, chopped
- 1 tsp.. flax seeds
- Salt and pepper, to taste

Directions:
1. Prepare the chickpeas and kidney beans according to the method. Soak the flax seeds according to the method, and then drain excess water.
2. Prepare the dressing by adding the basil, olive oil, lemon juice, salt, and half of the avocado to a food processor or blender. Pulse at low speed.
3. Continually, add small amounts of water until the dressing is creamy and smooth. Move the dressing to a small bowl and set it aside.
4. Combine the kale, Brussel sprouts, cooked chickpeas, kidney beans, radishes, walnuts, and remaining avocado in a large bowl and mix

thoroughly. Store the mixture, or serve with the dressing and flax seeds, and enjoy!

Nutrition: Calories: 266 kcal, Fat: 26.6 g, Saturated Fat: 5.1 g, Cholesterol: 0 mg, Sodium: 298 mg, Carbohydrate: 8.8 g, Dietary Fiber: 6.8 g, Sugars: 0.6 g, Protein: 2.0 g, Vitamin D: 0 mcg, Calcium: 19 mg, Iron: 1 mg, Potassium: 500 mg

141.   Sweet Potato & Black Bean Protein Salad

Preparation Time: 15 minutes, **Cooking Time:** 50 minutes, **Difficulty Level:** Hard, **Servings:** 4

Ingredients:
- 1 cup dry black beans
- 4 cups spinach
- 1 medium sweet potato
- 1 cup purple onion, chopped
- 2 Tbsp. olive oil
- 2 Tbsp. lime juice
- 1 Tbsp. minced garlic
- ½ Tbsp. chili powder
- ¼ tsp.. cayenne
- ¼ cup parsley
- ¼ tsp. Salt
- ¼ tsp. pepper

Directions:
1. Prepare the black beans according to the method. Preheat the oven to 400 °F.
2. Cut the sweet potato into ¼-inch cubes and put these in a medium-sized bowl. Add the onions, 1 tablespoon of olive oil, and salt to taste.
3. Toss the ingredients until the sweet potatoes and onions are completely coated. Transfer the ingredients to a baking sheet lined with parchment paper and spread them out in a single layer.
4. In the oven, place the baking sheet and roast until the sweet potatoes start to turn brown and crispy, around 40 minutes. Meanwhile, combine the remaining olive oil, lime juice, garlic, chili powder, and cayenne thoroughly in a large bowl until no lumps remain.
5. Remove the sweet potatoes and onions from the oven and transfer them to the large bowl. Add the cooked black beans, parsley, and a pinch of salt.
6. Toss everything until well combined. Then mix in the spinach and serve in desired portions with additional salt and pepper. Store or enjoy!

Nutrition: Calories: 558 kcal, Fat: 16.2 g, Saturated Fat: 2.5 g, Cholesterol: 0 mg, Sodium: 390 mg, Carbohydrate: 84.0 g, Dietary Fiber: 20.4 g, Sugars: 8.9 g, Protein: 25.3

g, Vitamin D: 0 mcg, Calcium: 220 mg, Iron: 10 mg, Potassium: 2243 mg

142. Taco Tempeh Salad

Preparation Time: 25 minutes, **Cooking Time:** 12 minutes, **Difficulty Level:** Moderate, **Servings:** 4

Ingredients:
- 1 cup dry black beans
- 1 8-oz. package tempeh
- 1 Tbsp.. lime or lemon juice
- 2 Tbsp.. extra virgin olive oil
- 1 tsp.. maple syrup
- ½ tsp. Chili powder
- ¼ tsp. cumin
- ¼ tsp. paprika
- 1 large bunch of kale, fresh or frozen, chopped
- 1 large avocado, peeled, pitted, diced
- ½ cup salsa
- ¼ tsp. salt
- ¼ tsp. pepper

Directions:
1. Prepare the beans according to the method.
2. Cut the tempeh into ¼-inch cubes, place in a bowl, and then add the lime or lemon juice, 1 tablespoon of olive oil, maple syrup, chili powder, cumin, and paprika.
3. Stir well and let the tempeh marinate in the fridge for at least 1 hour, up to 12 hours.
4. Over medium heat, warm the remaining olive oil in a frying pan.
5. Add the marinated tempeh mixture and cook until brown and crispy on both sides, around 10 minutes.
6. Put the chopped kale in a bowl with the cooked beans and prepare tempeh.
7. Store, or serve the salad immediately, topped with salsa, avocado, and salt and pepper to taste.

Nutrition: Calories: 627 kcal, Fat: 31.7 g, Saturated Fat: 6.1 g, Cholesterol: 0 mg, Sodium: 493 mg, Carbohydrate: 62.7 g, Dietary Fiber: 16 g, Sugars: 4.5 g, Protein: 31.4 g, Vitamin D: 0 mcg, Calcium: 249 mg, Iron: 7 mg, Potassium: 1972mg

143. Tempeh "Chicken" Salad

Preparation Time: 10 minutes, **Cooking Time:** 0 minutes, **Difficulty Level:** Easy, **Servings:** 4

Ingredients:
- 4 Tbsp. light mayonnaise
- 2 scallions, sliced
- Pepper, to taste
- 4 cups mixed salad greens
- 4 tsp. white miso
- 2 Tbsp. chopped fresh dill
- 1 ½ cups crumbled tempeh
- 1 cup sliced grape tomatoes

Directions:
To Make the Dressing:
1. Add mayonnaise, scallions, miso, dill, and pepper into a bowl and whisk well.
2. Add tempeh and fold gently.
To Serve:
1. Divide the greens into 4 plates. Divide the tempeh among the plates. Top with tomatoes and serve.

Nutrition: Calories: 452 kcal, Fat: 24.5 g, Saturated Fat: 4.4 g, Cholesterol: 8 mg, Sodium: 733 mg, Carbohydrate: 37.2 g, Dietary Fiber: 2.6 g, Sugars: 5.3 g, Protein: 29.9 g, Vitamin D: 0 mcg, Calcium: 261 mg, Iron: 8 mg, Potassium: 1377 mg

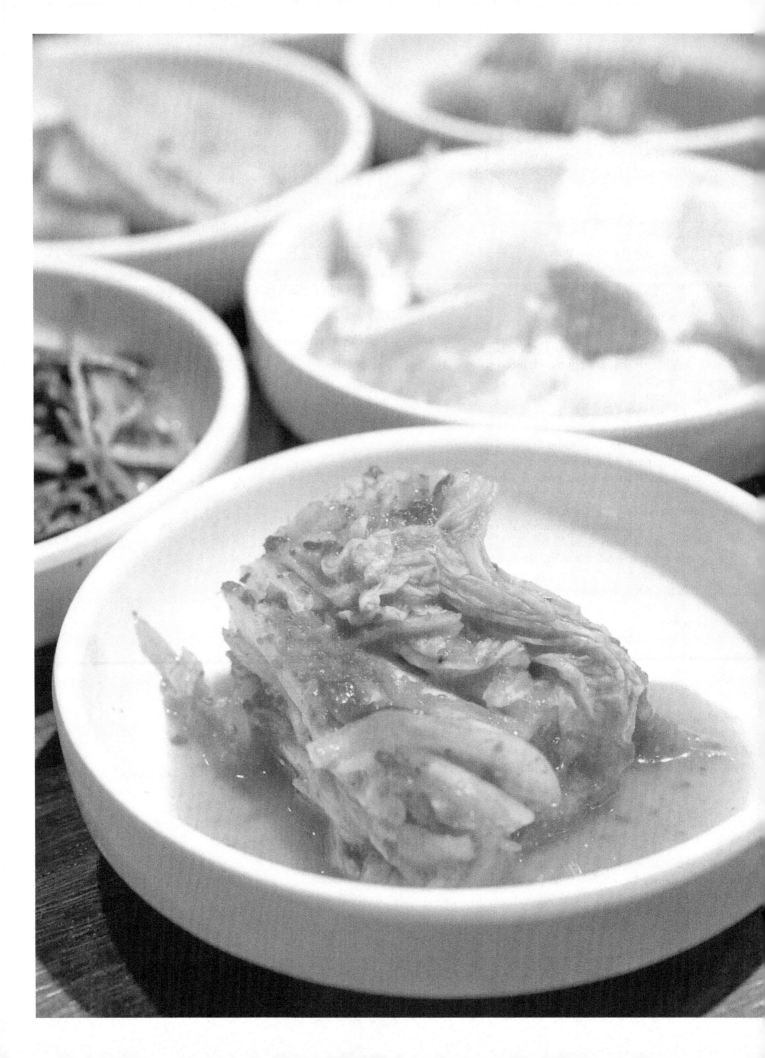

Chapter 12: Sides

144. Baked Beans with Mustard

Preparation Time: 5 minutes, **Cooking Time:** 15 minutes, **Difficulty Level:** Moderate, **Servings:** 4

Ingredients:

- ½ cup kidney beans rinsed and drained
- ½ cup pinto beans rinsed and drained
- ½ cup chickpea beans rinsed and drained
- 1 cup water
- ½ cup tomato paste
- 1 tsp. honey
- ½ Tbsp. ground mustard
- 1 tsp. paprika

Directions:

1. Add the kidney beans, pinto beans, chickpeas beans, water, tomato paste, honey, ground mustard, and paprika. Lock the lid, turn the valve to "Sealing" mode, then select Manual or Pressure Cook and adjust the pressure to High.
2. Set the Time for 8 minutes. When cooking ends, let the pressure release naturally for 15 minutes, then turn the valve to "Venting" to quickly release the pressure remaining. Unlock, remove the lid, and stir well before serving.

Nutrition: Calories: 268 kcal, Fat: 2.7 g, Saturated Fat: 0.3 g, Cholesterol: 0 mg, Sodium: 555 mg, Carbohydrate: 50.6 g, Dietary Fiber: 13.0 g, Sugars: 11.8 g, Protein: 14.0 g

145. Cinnamon Carrots

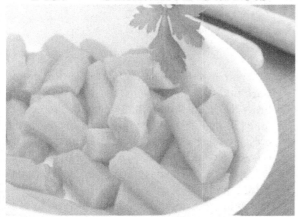

Preparation Time: 10 minutes, **Cooking Time:** 15 minutes, **Difficulty Level:** Easy, **Servings:** 4

Ingredients:

- 1 lb. baby carrots, scrubbed
- ⅓ cup water
- 1 tsp. ground cinnamon
- ¼ tsp. chili powder
- 1 tsp. black pepper

Directions:

1. In the instant pot, mix the carrots with the water and the other ingredients. Close the lid and Manual mode (High pressure) for 15 minutes.
2. After this, use quick pressure release.
3. Divide between plates and serve.

Nutrition: Calories: 147 kcal, Fat: 0.5 g, Fiber: 7.1 g, Carbs: 9.9 g, Protein: 4.3 g

146. Easy Lentil and Vegetable Curry

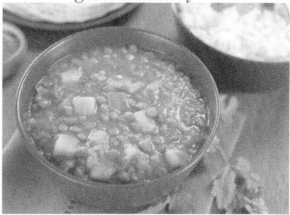

Preparation Time: 10 minutes, **Cooking Time:** 45 minutes, **Difficulty Level:** Moderate, **Servings:** 4

Ingredients:

- 3 ½ cups water
- ½ Tbsp. butter
- ¼ tsp. cumin seeds
- ½ tsp. coriander seeds
- ¼ tsp. turmeric powder
- ¼ tsp. paprika
- ½ tsp. garam masala
- ½ tsp. garlic powder
- ¼ tsp. ginger powder
- ¼ cup onion, finely chopped
- 2 cups chopped veggies of your choice (red pepper, carrot, cabbage, broccoli, etc.
- ¼ cup dried red lentils
- 1 ½ cups vegetable stock
- ½ full-fat milk
- ¼ cup green peas
- 1 tsp. lime juice
- ¼ tsp. of sea salt

- ¼ tsp. ground pepper

Directions:
1. Select the setting of High Sauté on the Instant Pot and heat the butter. Add the cumin seeds directly to the melted butter at the bottom edges of the Instant Pot. Cook until the ingredients start to sizzle, about 1 minute.
2. Add the onion and cook, occasionally stirring, until translucent, about 5 minutes. Add the ginger powder and garlic powder and sauté until aromatic, about 1 minute. Add the coriander seeds, salt, paprika, turmeric powder, chopped vegetables, and red lentils; pour in the 1 ½ cups water, and stir properly.
3. Secure the lid. Set the Pressure Release to Seal. Press Cancel to reset the cooking program, select Pressure Cook or Manual, and set the cooking time for 35 minutes at High Pressure.
4. Let the pressure release naturally. Note, this may take up to 10 to 20 minutes. Open the Instant Pot and stir in the green peas and garam masala milk. Select the High Sauté setting and cook for 2 minutes. To turn off the Instant Pot, press the Cancel button. Ladle into bowls, sprinkle with the cilantro and lime juice, serve.

Nutrition: Calories: 200 kcal, Fat: 4.2 g, Saturated Fat: 2.4 g, Cholesterol: 8 mg, Sodium: 331 mg, Carbohydrate: 31.3 g, Dietary Fiber: 11.9 g, Sugars: 5.8 g, Protein: 9.8 g

147.   Fava Beans

Preparation Time: 15 minutes, **Cooking Time:** 30 minutes, **Difficulty Level:** Moderate, **Servings:** 4

Ingredients:
- 1 tsp. olive oil
- 1 small onion, chopped
- 1 tomato, chopped
- 1 Tbsp. tomato paste
- 1 cup of water
- ½ cup fava beans, drained
- ½ Tbsp. ground cumin
- ½ tsp. salt
- 1 ½ tsp. ground black pepper
- ½ tsp. ground red pepper
- 1 Tbsp. finely chopped parsley

Directions:
1. In your Instant Pot, sauté olive oil and add onions. Cook and stir for 2 minutes. Add chopped tomatoes and tomato paste; cook until tomatoes are mushy, about 4 minutes.
2. Pour fava beans into Instant Pot. Add 1 cup water, cumin, salt, black pepper, and ground red pepper; stir well. Close the lid to seal the vent Instant Pot.

Set the cooker for 23 minutes and cook at High pressure on the Manual setting.
3. Release the pressure naturally.
4. Stir in parsley.

Nutrition: Calories: 186 kcal, Fat: 3.5 g, Saturated Fat: 0.5 g, Cholesterol: 0 mg, Sodium: 602 mg, Carbohydrate: 29.9 g, Dietary Fiber: 11.6 g, Sugars:5.5 g, Protein:11.4 g

148.   Garbanzo Beans with Kale

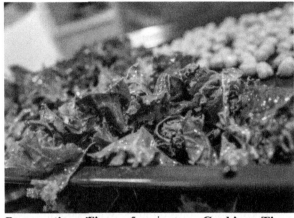

Preparation Time: 5 minutes, **Cooking Time:** 30 minutes, **Difficulty Level:** Moderate, **Servings:** 4

Ingredients:
- ½ cup dried garbanzo beans rinsed
- 2 cups of water
- ½ cup tomato paste
- ¼ tsp. garlic powder
- ¼ tsp. ginger powder
- ½ Tbsp. curry powder
- ¼ tsp. cinnamon powder
- ¼ tsp. salt
- ¼ tsp. ground black pepper
- 2 cups fresh kale

Directions:
1. Add garbanzo beans and water to the Instant Pot. Lock lid.
2. Press the beans button and cook for the default time (30 minutes). When the Timer beeps, let the pressure release naturally for 10 minutes. Quick-release any additional pressure until the float valve drops and then unlock the lid. Drain any extra liquid.
3. Stir in the remaining ingredients. Switch to Low Pressure and simmer for 4 minutes to heat through and wilt kale.
4. Move the mixture to a serving dish and serve warm.

Nutrition: Calories: 129 kcal, Fat: 1.8 g, Saturated Fat: 0.1 g, Cholesterol: 0 mg, Sodium: 395 mg, Carbohydrate: 26.6 g, Dietary Fiber: 6.1 g, Sugars: 8.1 g, Protein: 7.1 g

149.   Herbed Lentil Chili

Preparation Time: 10 minutes, **Cooking Time:** 20 minutes, **Difficulty Level:** Moderate, **Servings:** 4

Ingredients:
- 1 Tbsp. coconut oil
- 1 small onion chopped
- ½ tsp. garlic powder
- 1 zucchini chopped
- 1 leek chopped
- ½ Tbsp. paprika
- ¼ tsp. cumin powder
- ¼ tsp. coriander powder
- ½ tsp. dried basil
- ¼ tsp. dry mustard
- 1 cup crushed tomatoes
- ½ cup dry lentils
- 1 ½ cups low sodium vegetable broth
- Salt to taste
- ¼ tsp. pepper

Directions:
1. Select the "Sauté" setting on Instant Pot. Add coconut oil and let heat up. Add onions, garlic powder, zucchinis, and leeks.
2. Sauté until onions are softened and lightly browned, about 4 minutes. Add paprika, cumin powder, coriander powder, basil, mustard, and stir well for a minute or two. Add tomatoes, lentils, broth, salt to taste, and pepper.
3. Select "Cancel," then close the lid. Turn steam release handle to "Sealing" position. Select "Bean/Chili" and set the timer for 14 minutes.
4. Press "Cancel" and let Instant Pot naturally release pressure until the float valve drops down and lid unlocks; alternatively, press "Cancel" and let Instant Pot naturally release for 10 minutes. Turn steam release valve to "Venting" until float valve drops down and lid unlocks.

Nutrition: Calories: 296 kcal, Calories from Fat: 27 kcal, Fat: 3.0 g, Sodium: 596 mg, Potassium: 935 mg, Carbohydrates: 49 g, Fiber: 22 g, Sugar: 6 g, Protein: 18 g

150.   Kale Polenta

Preparation Time: 5 minutes, **Cooking Time:** 8 minutes, **Difficulty Level:** Moderate, **Servings:** 4

Ingredients:
- 1 cup polenta
- ½ cup kale, chopped
- 1 tsp. turmeric powder
- 1 tsp. smoked paprika
- 4 cups vegetable broth
- 2 Tbsp. coconut milk
- ½ tsp. ground black pepper
- 1 tsp. salt

Directions:
1. Whisk together polenta and vegetable broth.
2. Pour mixture in the instant pot, add the rest of the ingredients, and toss.
3. Close the lid and cook it on Manual mode (High pressure) for 8 minutes. Use quick pressure release.
4. Transfer cooked polenta in the bowl, stir and serve.

Nutrition: Calories: 182 kcal, Fat: 2.8 g, Fiber: 1.0 g, Carbs: 20.5 g, Protein: 6.3 g

151.   Paprika Sweet Potato

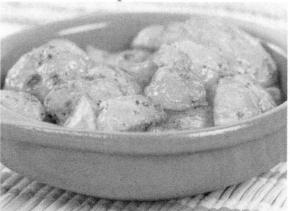

Preparation Time: 10 minutes, **Cooking Time:** 11 minutes, **Difficulty Level:** Moderate, **Servings:** 4

Ingredients:
- 2 sweet potatoes
- 2 tsp. sweet paprika
- ½ tsp. oregano, dried
- 1 tsp. chili powder
- 1 tsp. chives, chopped
- ½ cup of water

Directions:
1. In the instant pot, pour water and insert steamer rack.
2. Put potatoes on the rack and close the lid.
3. Set Manual mode (High pressure) and cook for 11 minutes. Then use quick pressure release.
4. Transfer the potatoes to the plate, cut them into halves, sprinkle the ingredients on top, and serve.

Nutrition: Calories: 159 kcal, Fat: 3.4 g, Fiber: 2.8 g, Carbs: 33.8 g, Protein: 3.6 g

152.   Potato Mash

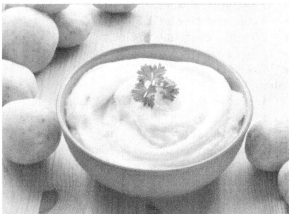

Preparation Time: 10 minutes, **Cooking Time:** 9 minutes, **Difficulty Level:** Easy, **Servings:** 4

Ingredients:
- 1 ½ lb. white potatoes, peeled and chopped
- 1 tsp. salt
- ½ tsp. hot paprika
- 1 tsp. dill, dried
- 1 Tbsp. coconut butter
- 1 tsp. ground black pepper
- 1 cup vegetable broth
- 1 Tbsp. fresh parsley, chopped

Directions:
1. Put potatoes, salt, and vegetable broth in the instant pot.
2. Close the lid and set manual mode. Cook on High for 9 minutes.
3. Then make a quick pressure release, strain the sweet potatoes and mash until smooth.
4. Add the rest of the ingredients. Stir properly before serving.

Nutrition: Calories: 123 kcal, Fat: 4.3 g, Fiber: 2.2 g, Carbs: 11.4 g, Protein: 4.3 g

153.   Red Cabbage and Carrots

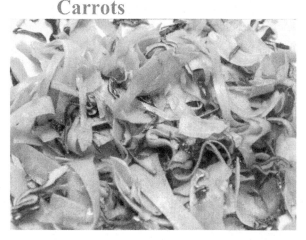

Preparation Time: 10 minutes, **Cooking Time:** 7 minutes, **Difficulty Level:** Easy, **Servings:** 4

Ingredients:
- 1 lb. red cabbage, shredded
- 2 carrots, peeled and grated
- 1 tsp. turmeric powder
- 1 tsp. coriander, ground
- 1 tsp. black pepper
- 1 tsp. salt
- ¼ cup of coconut milk
- ¾ cup almond milk
- ½ Tbsp. chives, chopped

Directions:
1. In the instant pot, mix the cabbage with the carrots and the other ingredients. Toss and set manual mode (High pressure).
2. Cook the cabbage for 7 minutes. Then allow natural pressure release.
3. Transfer the meal into the serving bowls and cool down before serving

Nutrition: Calories: 182 kcal, Fat: 5.1 g, Fiber: 3.4 g, Carbs: 12.3 g, Protein: 2.6 g

154.   Rosemary Lentils, Beans Curry

Preparation Time: 10 minutes, **Cooking Time:** 30 minutes, **Difficulty Level:** Moderate, **Servings:** 4

Ingredients:
- 1 cup of water
- ½ cup of brown rice
- ½ cup brown lentils
- ½ cup navy beans pre-soaked or quick-soaked
- ½ Tbsp. rosemary
- 1 tsp. garlic powder
- ½ cup chopped onions
- ½ cup low-sodium vegetable broth

Directions:
1. In your Instant Pot, sauté the onions in the vegetable broth and garlic powder. First, heat the broth on medium and sauté the onion for about 4 minutes until translucent, then add the garlic powder for another 30 seconds.
2. Add the rest of the ingredients to Instant Pot and stir properly.
3. Close the lid to seal the vent of the instant pot. For 23 minutes, set the cooker and cook at high pressure on the manual setting.
4. Release the pressure naturally.
5. Serve and season as desired.

Nutrition: Calories: 269 kcal, Fat: 1.6 g, Saturated Fat: 0.3 g, Cholesterol: 0 mg,Sodium: 255 mg, Carbohydrate: 55.2 g, Dietary Fiber: 7.4 g, Sugars: 1.6 g, Protein: 9.9 g

155. Spinach Split Pigeon Pea

Preparation Time: 15 minutes, **Cooking Time:** 15 minutes, **Difficulty Level:** Moderate, **Servings:** 4

Ingredients:
- ½ cup split pigeon pea
- 1 cup spinach chopped
- ½ Tbsp. vegetable oil
- ¼ tsp. cumin seeds
- 1 green chili pepper sliced (optional)
- ¼ tsp. ginger powder
- ½ tsp. garlic powder
- 1 tomato large, chopped
- 2 cups of water
- ¼ tsp. garam masala
- ¼ tsp. salt
- ⅛ tsp. turmeric powder
- ¼ tsp. red chili powder

Directions:
1. Start the Instant Pot in Sauté mode and heat vegetable oil in it. Add cumin seeds, green chili, ginger powder, and garlic powder.
2. Sauté for 30 seconds until garlic turns golden brown, then add chopped tomatoes and spices.
3. Add the split pigeon pea and water, then stir properly. Press Cancel and close the Instant Pot lid with the vent in the Sealing position.
4. For 3 minutes, Press Manual or Pressure Cook mode. Do a Quick Pressure Release when the Instant Pot beeps.
5. Open the lid. Add chopped spinach and garam masala. Press Sauté. Simmer for 2 minutes until the dal starts boiling, and spinach is mixed with the lentils.
6. Spinach split pigeon pea is ready to be served.

Nutrition: Calories: 240 kcal, Fat: 4. 8 g, Saturated Fat: 1.0 g, Cholesterol: 0 mg, Sodium: 325 mg, Carbohydrate: 38.8 g, Dietary Fiber: 4.5 g, Sugars: 5.8 g, Protein: 13.4 g

156. Three-Lentil Curry

Preparation Time: 10 minutes **Cooking Time:** 25 minutes **Difficulty Level:** Hard, **Servings:** 4

Ingredients:
- ½ Tbsp. coconut oil
- 1 tsp. garlic powder
- 1 tsp. ginger powder
- ½ Tbsp. garam masala

- 1 tsp. cumin powder
- ¼ tsp. turmeric powder
- ¼ tsp. table salt
- ¼ tsp. paprika
- 1 cinnamon stick 4-inch stick
- 2 green cardamom pods
- 1 bay leaf
- ½ cup red tomatoes chopped
- ¼ cup red lentils
- ¼ cup brown lentils
- ¼ cup green lentils
- ¼ cup
- 4 cups of water
- ½ cup coconut cream

Directions:
1. Press Sauté set the Time for 5 minutes.
2. Add coconut oil to the Instant Pot. Add the garlic powder, ginger powder, garam masala, cumin powder, turmeric powder, salt, paprika, cinnamon stick, cardamom pods, and bay leaves. Stir until fragrant, about 1 minute. Add the tomatoes and cook, often stirring, until it just begins to break down, 1 to 2 minutes.
3. Turn off the Sauté function. Stir the red lentils, brown lentils, and green lentils until well coated in spices. Then stir in the water and lock the lid of the Instant Pot.
4. For 16 minutes, Press Pressure Cook on Max Pressure with the Keep Warm setting off.
5. Use the Quick-release method to bring the Instant Pot pressure back to normal. Unlatch the lid, open the Instant Pot, and remove the cardamom pods, cinnamon sticks, and bay leaves. Then, stir in the cream until uniform, and set the lid askew over the Instant Pot for 5 minutes to blend the flavors. Stir again before serving.

Nutrition: Calories: 340 kcal, Fat: 21. 1 g, Saturated Fat: 16.3 g, Cholesterol: 0 mg, Sodium: 390 mg, Carbohydrate: 30.8 g, Dietary Fiber: 10.8 g, Sugars: 5.7 g, Protein: 10.4 g

157. Marinated Mushrooms

Preparation Time: 15 minutes, **Cooking Time:** 25 minutes, **Difficulty Level:** Moderate, **Servings:** 4

Ingredients:
- 1 cup red wine
- ½ cup red wine vinegar
- ⅓ cup olive oil
- 2 Tbsp. brown sugar
- 2 cloves garlic, minced
- 1 tsp. crushed red pepper flakes
- ¼ cup red bell pepper, diced

- 1 lb. small fresh mushrooms, washed and trimmed
- ¼ cup chopped green onions
- ¼ tsp. dried oregano
- ½ tsp. salt
- ¼ tsp. ground black pepper

Directions:
1. Mix the mushrooms, red pepper flakes, bell pepper, garlic, sugar, oil, vinegar, and wine in a saucepan on medium heat, then boil.
2. Put the cover and put it aside to let it cool.
3. Mix in pepper, salt, oregano, and green onions once cooled. Serve it at room temperature or chilled.

Nutrition: Calories: 135 kcal, Fat: 5.0 g, Carbs: 13.0 g, Protein: 8.0 g

158.   Low-fat Stuffed Mushrooms

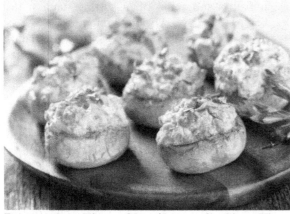

Preparation Time: 20 minutes, **Cooking Time:** 25 minutes, **Difficulty Level:** Moderate, **Servings:** 4

Ingredients:
- 1 lb. large fresh mushrooms
- 3 Tbsp. seasoned breadcrumbs
- 3 Tbsp. fat-free sour cream
- 2 Tbsp. grated Parmesan cheese
- 2 tsp. balsamic vinegar
- 2 Tbsp. minced chives
- 2 to 3 drops hot pepper sauce, optional
- 2 Tbsp. reduced-fat mayonnaise

Directions:
1. Take out the stems from the mushrooms, then put the cups aside. Chop the stems and set aside ⅓ cup (get rid of the leftover stems or reserve for later use).
2. Mix the reserved mushroom stems, hot pepper sauce if preferred, vinegar, mayonnaise, chives,

Parmesan cheese, sour cream, and breadcrumbs in a bowl, then stir well.
3. Put the mushroom caps on a cooking spray-coated baking tray and stuff it with the crumb mixture.
4. For 5 to 7 minutes, let it boil placed 4-6 inches from the heat source, or until it turns light brown.

Nutrition: Calories: 435 kcal, Fat: 4.0 g, Carbs: 23.0 g, Protein: 9.0 g

159.   Italian Stuffed Artichokes

Preparation Time: 20 minutes, **Cooking Time:** 25 minutes, **Difficulty Level:** Hard, **Servings:** 4

Ingredients:
- 4 large artichokes
- 2 tsp. lemon juice
- 2 cups soft Italian breadcrumbs, toasted
- ½ cup grated Parmigiano-Reggiano cheese
- ½ cup minced fresh parsley
- 2 tsp. Italian seasoning
- 1 tsp. grated lemon peel
- ½ tsp. pepper
- ¼ tsp. salt
- 1 Tbsp. olive oil

Directions:
1. Level the bottom of each artichoke using a sharp knife and trim off 1-inch from the tops. Snip off tips of outer leaves using kitchen scissors, then brush lemon juice on cut edges. In a Dutch oven, stand the artichokes and pour 1-inch of water, then boil. Lower the heat, put the cover, and let it simmer for 5 minutes or until the leaves near the middle pull out effortlessly.
2. Turn the artichokes upside down to the drain. Allow it to stand for 10 minutes. Carefully scrape out the fuzzy middle part of the artichokes using a spoon and get rid of it.
3. Mix the salt, pepper, lemon peel, Italian seasoning, garlic, parsley, cheese, and breadcrumbs in a small bowl, add olive oil and stir well. Gently spread the artichoke leaves apart, then fill it with breadcrumb mixture.
4. Now spray an 11x7-inch baking dish with cooking spray and place artichokes. Let it bake for 10 minutes at 350 °F without cover or until the filling turns light brown.

Nutrition: Calories: 543 kcal, Fat: 5.0 g, Carbs: 44.0 g, Protein: 6.0 g

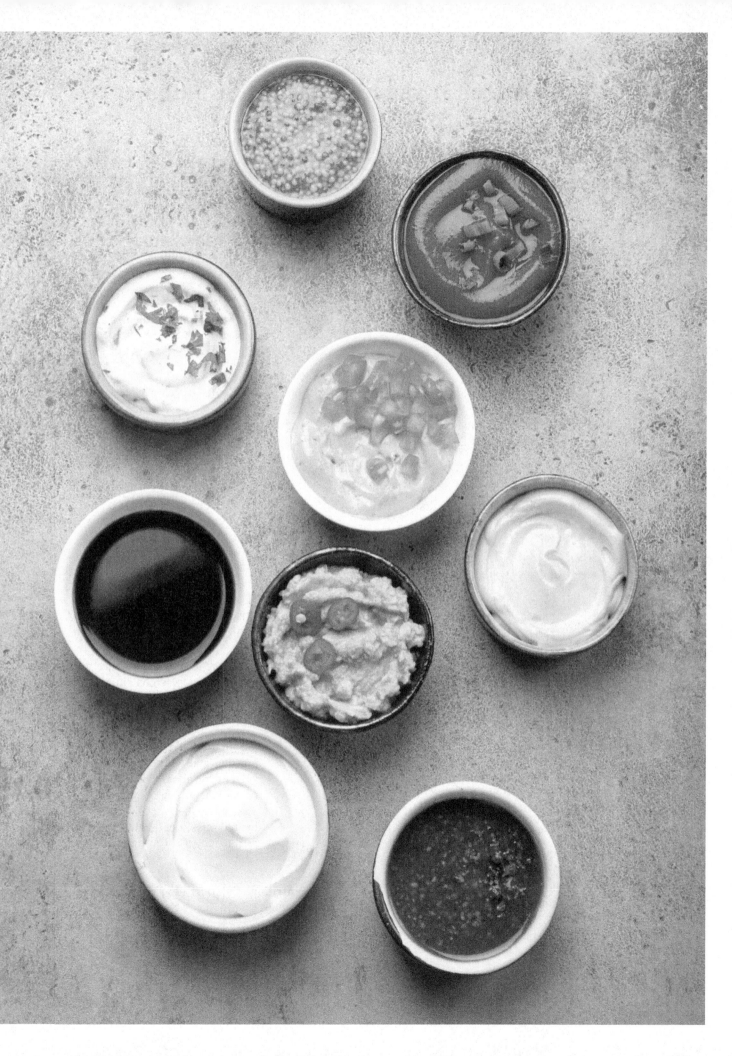

Chapter 13: Sauces, Dips, and Condiments

160.   Avocado Hummus

Preparation Time: 5 minutes, **Cooking Time:** 5 minutes, **Difficulty Level:** Easy, **Servings:** 4

Ingredients:
- 1 Tbsp.. cilantro, finely chopped
- ⅛ t. cumin
- 1 garlic clove
- 3 Tbsp.. lime juice
- 1 ½ Tbsp. tahini
- 1 ½ Tbsp. olive oil
- 2 avocados, medium cored & peeled
- 15 oz. chickpeas, drained
- Salt and pepper to taste

Directions:
1. In a food processor, add garlic, lime juice, tahini, olive oil, and chickpeas and pulse until combined.
2. Add cumin and avocados and blend until smooth consistency, approximately 2 minutes.
3. Add salt and pepper to taste.

Nutrition: Calories: 310 kcal, Carbohydrates: 26.0 g, Proteins: 8.0 g, Fats: 20.0 g

161.   Beans Mayonnaise

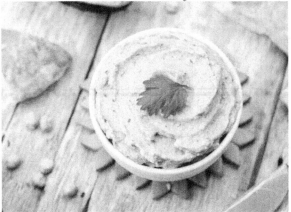

Preparation Time: 10 minutes, **Cooking Time:** 2 minutes, **Difficulty Level:** Easy, **Servings:** 4

Ingredients:
- 2 Tbsp. apple cider vinegar
- 1 Tbsp. fresh lemon juice
- 2 Tbsp. yellow mustard
- 1 (15- oz.) can of white beans, drained and rinsed
- ¾ tsp. salt
- 2 Tbsp. aquafaba (liquid from the can of beans)
- 2 garlic cloves, peeled

- ⅔ cups olive oil

Directions:
1. In a food processor, add all ingredients (except for oil) and pulse until mostly pureed.
2. While the motor is running, add the reserved oil and pulse until light and smooth.
3. Transfer the mayonnaise into a container and refrigerate to chill before serving.

Nutrition: Calories: 8 kcal, Fat: 1.1 g, Saturated Fat: 0.1 g, Cholesterol: 0 mg, Sodium: 559 mg, Carbs: 14.3 g, Fiber: 4.1 g, Sugar: 0.2 g, Protein: 5.2 g

162.   Beer "Cheese" Dip

Preparation Time: 10 minutes, **Cooking Time:** 7 minutes, **Difficulty Level:** Moderate, **Servings:** 4

Ingredients:
- ¾ cup water
- ¾ cup brown ale
- ½ cup raw cashews, soaked in hot water for at least 15 minutes, then drained
- 2 Tbsp. tomato paste
- ½ cup raw walnuts, soaked in hot water for at least 15 minutes, then drained
- 2 Tbsp. fresh lemon juice
- 1 Tbsp. apple cider vinegar
- ½ cup nutritional yeast
- ½ tsp. sweet or smoked paprika
- 1 Tbsp. arrowroot powder
- 1 Tbsp. red miso

Directions:
1. Place the water, brown ale, walnuts, cashews, tomato paste, lemon juice, and apple cider vinegar into a high-speed blender, and purée until thoroughly mixed and smooth.
2. Transfer to a saucepan over medium heat. Add the nutritional yeast, paprika, and arrowroot powder, and whisk well. Bring the mixture to a simmer for about 7 minutes, stirring frequently, or until the mixture begins to thicken and bubble.
3. Take away the saucepan from the heat. Whisk in the red miso. Let the dip cool for 10 minutes and refrigerate in an airtight container for up to 5 days.

Nutrition: Calories: 113 kcal, Fat: 5.1 g, Carbs: 10.4 g, Protein: 6.3 g, Fiber: 3.8 g

163. Cashew Cream

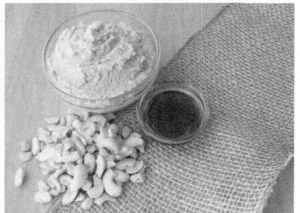

Preparation Time: 10 minutes, **Cooking Time:** 0 minutes, **Difficulty Level:** Easy, **Servings:** 4

Ingredients:
- 1 cup raw, unsalted cashews, soaked for 12 hours, and drained
- ½ cup water
- 1 Tbsp. nutritional yeast
- 1 tsp. fresh lemon juice
- ⅛ tsp. salt

Directions:
1. In a food processor, add all ingredients and pulse at high speed until creamy and smooth.
2. Serve immediately.

Nutrition: Calories: 165 kcal, Fat: 12.8 g, Saturated Fat: 2.5 g, Cholesterol: 0 mg, Sodium: 65 mg, Carbs: 9.9 g, Fiber: 1.3 g, Sugar: 1.4 g, Protein: 5.1 g

164. Chunky Cucumber Salsa

Preparation Time: 20 minutes, **Cooking Time:** 20 minutes, **Difficulty Level:** Easy, **Servings:** 4

Ingredients:
- 3 medium cucumbers, peeled and coarsely chopped
- 1 medium mango, coarsely chopped
- 1 cup frozen corn, thawed
- 1 medium sweet red pepper, coarsely chopped
- 1 small red onion, coarsely chopped
- 1 jalapeno pepper, finely chopped
- 3 garlic cloves, minced
- 2 Tbsp. white wine vinegar
- 1 Tbsp. minced fresh cilantro
- 1 tsp. salt
- ½ tsp. sugar
- ¼ to ½ tsp. cayenne pepper

Directions:
1. In a big bowl, mix all ingredients, then chill, covered, about 2 to 3 hours before serving.

Nutrition: Calories: 215 kcal, Fat: 5.0 g, Carbs: 23.0 g, Protein: 10.0 g

165. Healthier Guacamole

Preparation Time: 10 minutes, **Cooking Time:** 10 minutes, **Difficulty Level:** Easy, **Servings:** 4

Ingredients:
- ¾ cup crumbled tofu
- 2 avocados, peeled, pitted, and divided
- 1 tsp. salt
- 1 tsp. minced garlic
- 1 pinch cayenne pepper (optional)

Directions:
1. Prepare a food processor, put one avocado and tofu in it, and blend well until it becomes smooth. Combine salt, lime juice, and the left avocado in a bowl.
2. Add in the garlic, tomatoes, cilantro, onion, and tofu-avocado mixture. Put in cayenne pepper.
3. Let the guacamole chill in the refrigerator for 1 hour to enhance the flavor, or you can serve it right away.

Nutrition: Calories: 534 kcal, Fat: 5.0 g, Carbs: 23.0 g, Protein: 11.0 g

166. Creamy Black Bean Dip

Preparation Time: 10 minutes, **Cooking Time:** 0 minutes, **Difficulty Level:** Moderate, **Servings:** 4

Ingredients:
- ¼ tsp. salt (optional)
- 2 Tbsp. minced garlic
- 4 cups cooked black beans, rinsed and drained
- 2 Tbsp. low-sodium vegetable broth
- 1 Tbsp. lemon juice, or more to taste
- 2 Tbsp. Italian seasoning
- 2 Tbsp. onion powder

Directions:
1. In a large bowl, mash the black beans with a potato masher or the back of a fork until mostly smooth.
2. Add the other remaining ingredients to the bowl and whisk to combine.
3. Taste and add more lemon juice or salt, if needed. You can serve this immediately or refrigerate for at least 30 minutes to better incorporate the flavors.

Nutrition: Calories: 387 kcal, Fat: 6.5 g, Carbs: 63.0 g, Protein: 21.2 g, Fiber: 16.0 g

167. Easy Lemon Tahini Dressing

Preparation Time: 5 minutes, **Cooking Time:** 0 minutes, **Difficulty Level:** Easy, **Servings:** 4

Ingredients:
- ½ cup tahini
- ¼ cup fresh lemon juice (about 2 lemons)
- 1 tsp. maple syrup
- 1 small garlic clove, chopped
- ⅛ tsp. black pepper
- ¼ tsp. salt (optional)
- ¼ to ½ cup water

Directions:
1. Process the tahini, lemon juice, maple syrup, garlic, black pepper, and salt (if desired) in a blender (high-speed blenders work best for this). Slowly add the water until the mixture is completely smooth.
2. In an airtight container, store in the fridge for up to 5 days.

Nutrition: Calories: 128 kcal, Fat: 9.6 g, Carbs: 6.8 g, Protein: 3.6 g, Fiber: 1.9 g

168. Enchilada sauce

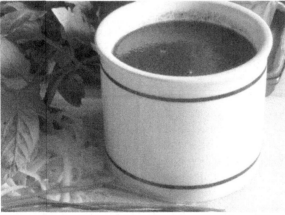

Preparation Time: 10 minutes, **Cooking Time:** 10 minutes, **Difficulty Level:** Moderate, **Servings:** 43

Ingredients:
- 1½ Tbsp. MCT oil
- ½ Tbsp. chili powder
- ½ Tbsp. whole wheat flour
- ½ tsp. ground cumin
- ¼ tsp. oregano (dried or fresh)
- ¼ tsp. salt (or to taste)
- 1 garlic clove (minced)

- 1 Tbsp. tomato paste
- 1 cup vegetable broth
- ½ tsp. apple vinegar
- ½ tsp. ground black pepper

Directions:
1. Heat a small saucepan over medium heat.
2. Add the MCT oil and minced garlic to the pan and sauté for about 1 minute.
3. Mix the dry spices and flour in a medium bowl and pour the dry mixture into the saucepan.
4. Stir in the tomato paste immediately, and slowly pour in the vegetable broth, ensuring that everything combines well.
5. When everything is mixed thoroughly, bring the heat to medium-high until it simmers. Cook for 3 minutes until the sauce becomes a bit thicker.
6. Remove from the heat and add the vinegar with the black pepper, adding more salt and pepper to taste.

Nutrition: Calories: 225 kcal, Fat: 4.0 g, Carbs: 33.0 g, Protein: 5.0 g

169. Fresh Mango Salsa

Preparation Time: 10 minutes, **Cooking Time:** 0 minutes, **Difficulty Level:** Easy, **Servings:** 4

Ingredients:
- 2 small mangoes, diced
- 1 red bell pepper, finely diced
- ½ red onion, finely diced
- ½ lime juice, or more to taste
- 2 Tbsp. low-sodium vegetable broth
- A handful of cilantro, chopped
- Freshly ground black pepper, to taste
- Salt, to taste (optional)

Directions:
1. Place all ingredients in a large bowl, and stir until well incorporated.
2. Taste and add more lime juice or salt; this is up to your preferred taste.
3. In an airtight container, store in the fridge for up to 5 days.

Nutrition: Calories: 86 kcal, Fat: 1.9 g, Carbs: 13.3 g, Protein: 1.2 g, Fiber: 0.9 g

170.   Garlic White Bean Dip

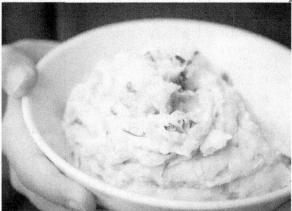

Preparation Time: 15 minutes, **Cooking Time:** 0 minute, **Difficulty Level:** Easy, **Servings:** 4

Ingredients:
- ¼ cup soft breadcrumbs
- 2 Tbsp. dry white wine or water
- 2 Tbsp. olive oil
- 2 Tbsp. lemon juice
- 4 ½ tsp.. minced fresh parsley
- 3 garlic cloves, peeled and halved
- ½ tsp. salt
- ½ tsp. snipped fresh dill or ¼ tsp. dill weed
- ⅛ tsp. cayenne pepper
- Assorted fresh vegetables

Directions:
1. Mix wine and breadcrumbs in a small bowl. Mix cayenne, dill, salt, garlic, parsley, beans, lemon juice, and oil in a food processor, then cover and blend until smooth.
2. Put in bread crumb mixture and process until well combined. Serve together with vegetables.

Nutrition: Calories: 105 kcal, Fat: 5.0 g, Carbs: 12.0 g, Protein: 6.0 g

171.   Guacamole

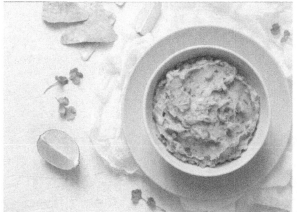

Preparation Time: 5 minutes, **Cooking Time:** 5 minutes, **Difficulty Level:** Moderate, **Servings:** 4

Ingredients:
- 3 Tbsp. tomato, diced
- 3 Tbsp. onion, diced
- 2 Tbsp. cilantro, chopped
- o juice
- ¼ tsp. garlic powder
- ½ tsp. salt
- ½ lime, squeezed
- 2 big avocados
- 1 Jalapeño, diced

Directions:
1. Using a molcajete, crush the diced jalapenos until soft.
2. Add the avocados to the molcajete.
3. Squeeze the lime juice from ½ of the lime on top of the avocados.
4. Add the Jalapeño juice, garlic, and salt and mix until smooth.
5. Once smooth, add in the onion, cilantro, and tomato and stir to incorporate.

Nutrition: Calories: 127 kcal, Carbohydrates: 9.3 g Proteins: 2.4 g, Fats: 10.2 g

172.   Homemade Tzatziki Sauce

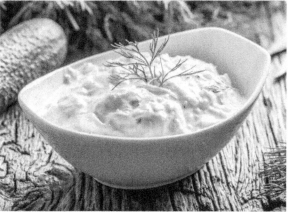

Preparation Time: 20 minutes, **Cooking Time:** 0 minutes, **Difficulty Level:** Easy, **Servings:** 4

Ingredients:
- 2 oz. (57 g) raw unsalted cashews (about ½ cup)
- 2 Tbsp. lemon juice
- ⅓ cup water
- 1 small clove of garlic
- 1 cup cucumber, peeled and chopped
- 2 Tbsp. fresh dill

Directions:

1. Add the cashews, water, lemon juice, and garlic to a blender. Keep it aside for at least 15 minutes to soften the cashews.
2. Blend the ingredients until smooth. Stir in the chopped cucumber and dill and continue to blend until it reaches your desired consistency. It doesn't need to be smooth. You're free to add more water if you like a thinner consistency.
3. Transfer to an airtight container and chill for at least 30 minutes for the best flavors.
4. Let the sauce cool to room temperature. Shake well before serving.

Nutrition: Calories: 208 kcal, Fat: 13.5 g, Carbs: 15.0 g, Protein: 6.7 g, Fiber: 2.8 g

173. Keto-Vegan Mayo

Preparation Time: 5 minutes, **Cooking Time:** 5 minutes, **Difficulty Level:** Easy, **Servings:** 4

Ingredients:
- ½ cup extra virgin olive oil
- ½ cup almond milk, unsweetened
- ¼ tsp. xanthan gum
- A pinch ground white pepper
- A pinch Himalayan salt
- 1 tsp. Dijon mustard
- 2 tsp. apple cider vinegar

Directions:

1. In a blender, place milk, pepper salt, mustard, and vinegar.
2. Set the blender to high speed. Slowly add xanthan, then the olive oil.
3. Remove from the blender and allow cooling for 2 hours in the refrigerator.
4. During cooling, the mixture will thicken.

Nutrition: Calories: 160.4, Carbohydrates: 0.2 g, Proteins: 0 g, Fats: 18 g

174. Lemon Tahini

Preparation Time: 15 minutes, **Cooking Time:** 0 minutes, **Difficulty Level:** Easy, **Servings:** 4

Ingredients:
- ¼ cup fresh lemon juice
- 4 medium garlic cloves, pressed
- ½ cup tahini
- ½ tsp. fine sea salt
- A pinch ground cumin
- 6 Tbsp. ice water

Directions:

1. Combine the lemon juice and garlic in a medium bowl and set aside for 10 minutes.
2. Through a fine-mesh sieve, strain the mixture into another medium bowl, pressing the garlic solids.
3. Discard the garlic solids.
4. In the bowl of lemon juice, add the tahini, salt, and cumin, and whisk until well blended.
5. Add water slowly, 2 Tbsp. at a time, whisking well after each addition.

Nutrition: Calories: 187 kcal, Fat: 16.3 g, Saturated Fat: 2.4 g, Cholesterol: 0 mg, Sodium: 273 mg, Carbs: 7.7 g, Fiber: 2.9 g, Sugar: 0.5 g, Protein: 5.4 g

175. Maple Dijon Dressing

Preparation Time: 5 minutes, **Cooking Time:** 0 minutes, **Difficulty Level:** Easy, **Servings:** 4

Ingredients:
- ¼ cup apple cider vinegar
- 2 tsp. Dijon mustard
- 2 Tbsp. maple syrup
- 2 Tbsp. low-sodium vegetable broth
- ¼ tsp. black pepper
- Salt, to taste (optional)

Directions:

- Mix the apple cider vinegar, Dijon mustard, maple syrup, vegetable broth, and black pepper in a resealable container until well incorporated. Season with salt to taste, if desired.
- This Maple Dijon dressing can be refrigerated for up to 5 days.

Nutrition: Calories: 82 kcal, Fat: 0.3 g, Carbs: 19.3 g, Protein: 0.6 g, Fiber: 0.7 g

176. Peanut Sauce

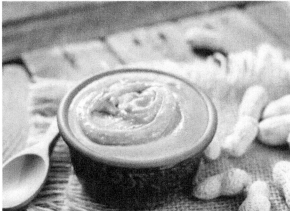

Preparation Time: 10 minutes, **Cooking Time:** 10 minutes, **Difficulty Level:** Moderate, **Servings:** 4

Ingredients:

- ½ tsp. Thai red curry paste
- 1 tsp. coconut oil
- 1 tsp. soy Sauce
- 1 tsp. chili garlic sauce
- 1 Tbsp. sweetener of your choice
- ⅓ cup coconut milk
- ¼ cup peanut butter, smooth

Directions:

1. Using a microwave-safe dish, add the peanut butter and heat for about 30 seconds.
2. Whisk into the peanut butter, soy sauce, sweetener, and chili garlic, then set to the side.
3. Warm a little saucepan over medium heat and add oil. Cook the Thai red curry paste until fragrant, then add to a microwave-safe bowl.
4. Continuously stir the peanut mixture as you add the coconut milk. Stir until well-combined.
5. Enjoy at room temperature or warmed.

Nutrition: Calories: 151 kcal, Carbohydrates: 4 g, Proteins: 4 g, Fats: 13 g

177. Pineapple Mint Salsa

Preparation Time: 10 minutes, **Cooking Time:** 0 minutes, **Difficulty Level:** Easy, **Servings:** 4

Ingredients:

- 1 lb. (454 g) fresh pineapple, finely diced, and juices reserved
- 1 bunch mint, leaves only, chopped
- 1 minced Jalapeño (optional)
- 1 white or red onion, finely diced
- Salt, to taste (optional)

Directions:

1. Mix the pineapple with its juice, mint, Jalapeño (if desired), and onion, and whisk well in a medium bowl. Season with salt to taste, if desired.
2. In an airtight container, refrigerate for at least 2 hours to better incorporate the flavors.

Nutrition: Calories: 58 kcal, Fat: 0.1 g, Carbs: 13.7 g Protein: 0.5 g, Fiber: 1.0 g

178. Pistachio Dip

Preparation Time: 10 minutes, **Cooking Time:** 10 minutes, **Difficulty Level:** Moderate, **Servings:** 4

Ingredients:

- 2 Tbsp. lemon juice
- 1 Tbsp. extra virgin olive oil
- 2 Tbsp. of the following:
- Tahini

- Parsley, chopped
- 2 garlic cloves
- ½ cup pistachios shelled
- 15 oz. garbanzo beans, with the liquid from the can
- Salt and pepper to taste

Directions:

1. Using a food processor, add pistachios, pepper, sea salt, lemon juice, olive oil, tahini, parsley, garlic, and garbanzo beans. Pulse until mixed.
2. Using the liquid from the garbanzo beans, add to the dip while slowly blending until it reaches your desired consistency.
3. Enjoy at room temperature or warmed.

Nutrition: Calories: 88 kcal, Carbohydrates: 9 g, Proteins: 2.5 g, Fats: 3.0 g

179. Pumpkin Spice Spread

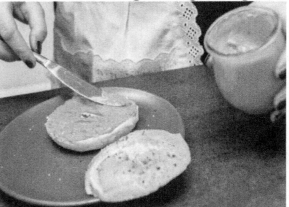

Preparation Time: 10 minutes, **Cooking Time:** 10 minutes, **Difficulty Level:** Moderate, **Servings:** 4

Ingredients:

- 1 package (8 oz.) fat-free cream cheese
- ½ cup canned pumpkin
- Sugar substitute equivalent to ½ cup sugar
- 1 tsp. ground cinnamon
- 1 tsp. vanilla extract
- 1 tsp. maple flavoring
- ½ tsp. pumpkin pie spice
- ½ tsp. ground nutmeg
- 1 carton (8 oz.) frozen reduced-fat whipped topping, thawed

Directions:

1. Mix well together sugar substitute, pumpkin, and cream cheese in a big bowl. Beat in nutmeg, pumpkin pie spice, maple flavoring, vanilla, and cinnamon.
2. Fold in whipped topping and chill until serving.

Nutrition: Calories: 177 kcal, Fat: 6.0 g, Carbs: 2.0 g, Protein: 11.0 g

180.   Smokey Tomato Jam

Preparation Time: 45 minutes, **Cooking Time:** 45 minutes, **Difficulty Level:** Moderate, **Servings:** 4 cups

Ingredients:
- ½ tsp. White wine vinegar
- ½ tsp. salt
- ⅓ t. smoked paprika
- A pinch of Black pepper
- ¼ cup coconut sugar
- 2 lb. tomatoes

Directions:
1. Boil a pot of water over medium-high heat. Fill a big bowl with ice and water.
2. Place the tomatoes carefully into the boiling water for 1 minute and then remove and immediately put into the ice water.
3. While tomatoes are in the ice water, peel them by hand and transfer them to a clean cutting surface. Empty the pot of water.
4. Chop the tomatoes and place back into the pot; add the coconut sugar and stir to combine.
5. Lower to medium heat and bring the tomatoes to a boil. Cook for 15 minutes.
6. Stir in the paprika, pepper, and salt, and then bring the temperature down to the lowest setting. Let it cook until it becomes thick, which is approximately 10 minutes.
7. Remove it from the heat while continuing to stir; add in white wine vinegar.

Nutrition: Calories: 26 kcal, Carbohydrates: 5.3 g Proteins: 1.1 g, Fats: 0.6 g

181.   Spicy and Tangy Black Bean Salsa

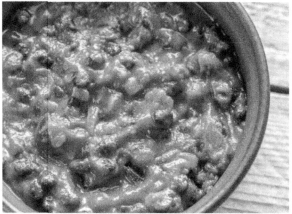

Preparation Time: 15 minutes, **Cooking Time:** 0 minutes, **Difficulty Level:** Easy, **Servings:** 4

Ingredients:
- 1 (15-oz. / 425-g) can cooked black beans, drained and rinsed
- 1 cup chopped tomatoes
- 1 cup corn kernels, thawed if frozen
- ½ cup cilantro or parsley, chopped
- ¼ cup finely chopped red onion
- 1 Tbsp. lemon juice
- 1 Tbsp. lime juice
- 1 tsp. chili powder
- ½ tsp. ground cumin
- ½ tsp. regular or smoked paprika
- 1 medium clove garlic, finely chopped

Directions:
1. In a large bowl, put all the ingredients and stir with a fork until well incorporated.
2. Serve immediately. You can also let it chill for 2 hours in the refrigerator to let the flavors blend.

Nutrition: Calories: 83 kcal, Fat: 0.5 g, Carbs: 15.4 g, Protein: 4.3 g, Fiber: 4.6 g

182.   Sweet Mango and Orange Dressing

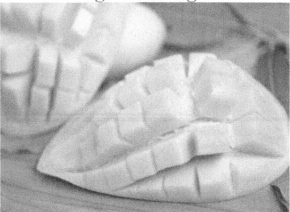

Preparation Time: 5 minutes, **Cooking Time:** 0 minutes, **Difficulty Level:** Easy, **Servings:** 4

Ingredients:
- 1 cup (165 g) diced mango, thawed if frozen
- ½ cup orange juice
- 2 Tbsp. rice vinegar
- 2 Tbsp. fresh lime juice
- ¼ tsp. salt (optional)
- 1 tsp. date sugar (optional)
- 2 Tbsp. chopped cilantro

Directions:

1. Pulse all the ingredients except for the cilantro in a food processor until it reaches the consistency you like. Add the cilantro and whisk well.
2. In an airtight container, store the dressing and keep it in the fridge for up to 2 days.

Nutrition: Calories: 32 kcal, Fat: 0.1 g, Carbs: 7.4 g, Protein: 0.3 g, Fiber: 0.5 g

183.   Tamari Vinegar Sauce

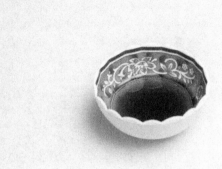

Preparation Time: 10 minutes, **Cooking Time:** 0 minutes, **Difficulty Level:** Easy, **Servings:** 4

Ingredients:
- ¼ cup tamari
- ½ cup nutritional yeast
- 2 Tbsp. balsamic vinegar
- 2 Tbsp. apple cider vinegar
- 2 Tbsp. Worcestershire sauce
- 2 tsp. Dijon mustard
- 1 Tbsp. + 1 tsp. maple syrup
- ½ tsp. ground turmeric
- ¼ tsp. black pepper

Directions:

1. Place all the ingredients in an airtight container, and whisk until everything is well incorporated.
2. Store in the refrigerator for up to 3 weeks.

Nutrition:
Calories: 216 kcal, Fat: 9.9 g, Carbs: 18.0 g, Protein: 13.7 g, Fiber: 7.7 g

184.   Tangy Cashew Mustard Dressing

Preparation Time: 20 minutes, **Cooking Time:** 0 minutes, **Difficulty Level:** Moderate, **Servings:** 4

Ingredients:

- 2 oz. (57 g) raw, unsalted cashews (about ½ cup)
- ½ cup water
- 3 Tbsp. lemon juice
- 2 tsp. apple cider vinegar
- 2 Tbsp. Dijon mustard
- 1 medium garlic clove

Directions:

1. In a food processor, put all the ingredients and keep them aside for at least 15 minutes.
2. Purée until the ingredients are combined into a smooth and creamy mixture. Thin the dressing with a little extra water as needed to achieve your preferred consistency.
3. In an airtight container, store the dressing and keep it in the refrigerator for up to 5 days.

Nutrition: Calories: 187 kcal, Fat: 13.0 g, Carbs: 11.5 g, Protein: 5.9 g, Fiber: 1.7 g

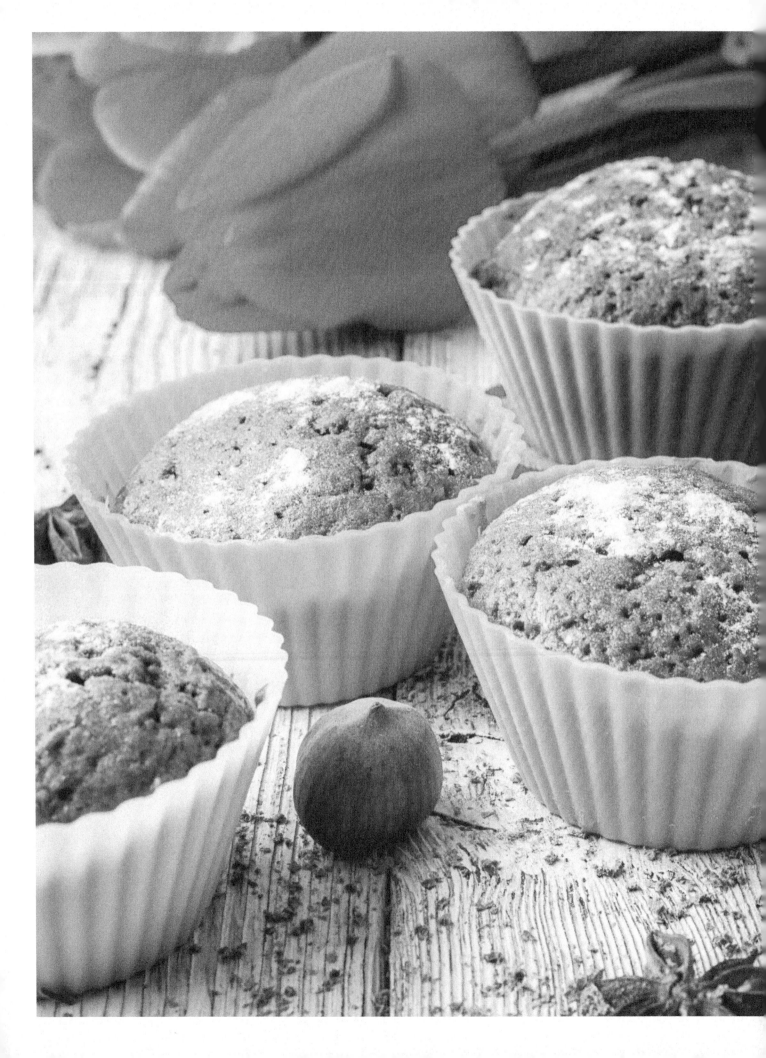

Chapter 14: Desserts and Sweets

185.   Almond Pulp Cookies

Preparation Time: 5 minutes, **Cooking Time:** 40 minutes, **Difficulty Level:** Hard, **Servings:** 4

Ingredients:
- 3 cups almond pulp
- 1 Granny Smith apple
- 1 to 2 tsp. cinnamon
- 2 to 3 Tbsp. raw honey
- ¼ cup coconut flakes

Directions:
- Blend almond pulp with remaining ingredients in a food processor. Make small cookies out of this mixture.
- On a cookie sheet that's lined with parchment paper, place the small cookies. Place the sheet in a food dehydrator for 6 to 10 hours at 115 °F. Serve.

Nutrition: Calories: 240 kcal, Fat: 22.5 g, Protein: 14.9 g

186.   Sautéed Pears

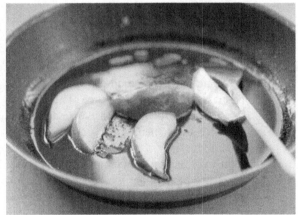

Preparation Time: 35 minutes, **Cooking Time:** 30 minutes, **Difficulty Level:** Moderate, **Servings:** 4

Ingredients:
- 2 Tbsp. Margarine (Or Vegan Butter)
- ¼ tsp. Cinnamon
- ¼ tsp. Nutmeg
- 6 Bosc Pears, Peeled & Quartered
- 1 Tbsp. Lemon Juice
- ½ Cup Walnuts, Toasted & Chopped (Optional)

Directions:
1. Melt your vegan butter in a skillet, and then add your spices. Cook for half a minute before adding in your pears.

2. Cook for fifteen minutes, and stir in your lemon juice.
3. Serve with walnuts if desired.

Interesting Facts:
Cinnamon is an absolute powerhouse and is considered one of the healthiest, beneficial spices on the plant. It's widely known for its medicinal properties. This spice is loaded with powerful antioxidants and is popular for its anti-inflammatory properties. It can reduce heart disease and lower blood sugar levels.

Nutrition: Calories: 189 kcal, Fat: 5.91 g, Protein: 0.78 g, Carbs: 33.39 g

187.   Fruit Skewers

Preparation Time: 20 minutes, **Cooking Time:** 20 minutes, **Difficulty Level:** Moderate, **Servings:** 4

Ingredients:
- 2 cups fresh/canned unsweetened pineapple chunks
- 1 cup cream cheese
- 1 cup sour cream
- 2 large red apples, cut into 1-inch pieces
- 2 tsp Lime juice
- ½ tsp. ground ginger
- Honey, to taste
- 2 cups green grapes

Directions:
1. To make the dip, beat the sour cream and cream cheese in a small bowl until it becomes smooth. Beat in the ginger, honey, and lime juice until it becomes smooth.
2. Put the cover and let it chill in the fridge for an hour minimum.
3. Alternately thread the apples, pineapple, and grapes on 8 12-inch skewers. Serve it right away with the dip.

Nutrition: Calories: 180 kcal, Fat: 5.0 g, Carbs: 28.0 g, Protein: 4.0 g

188.   Apple Almond Slush

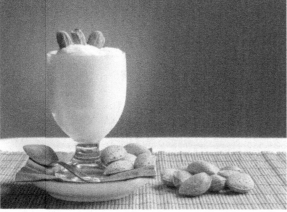

Preparation Time: 10 minutes, **Cooking Time:** 0 minutes, **Difficulty Level:** Easy, **Servings:** 4

Ingredients:
- 1 cup apple cider
- ½ cup coconut yogurt
- 4 Tbsp. almonds, crushed
- ¼ tsp. cinnamon
- ¼ tsp. nutmeg
- 1 cup ice cubes

Directions:
1.
2. Add all the ingredients to a blender.
3. Blend well until smooth. Serve.

Nutrition: Calories: 144 kcal, Fiber: 2.3 g, Protein: 5.6 g

189.   Avocado Pudding

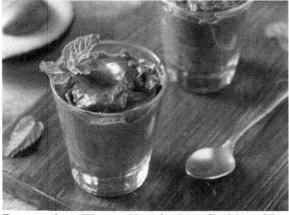

Preparation Time: 10 minutes, **Cooking Time:** 0 minutes, **Difficulty Level:** Easy, **Servings:** 4

Ingredients:
- 2 avocados
- ¾ to 1 cup almond milk
- ⅓-½ cup raw cacao powder
- 1 tsp. 100% pure organic vanilla (optional)
- 2 to 4 Tbsp. Swerve Sweetener

Directions:
1. Blend all the ingredients in a blender.
2. Refrigerate for 4 hours in a container. Serve.

Nutrition: Calories: 142 kcal, Fat: 9.5 g, Carbohydrates: 18 g, Protein: 3.52

190.   Banana Ice Cream

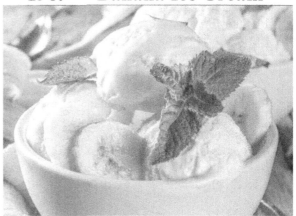

Preparation Time: 5 minutes, **Cooking Time:** 5 minutes, **Difficulty Level:** Easy, **Serving:** 4

Ingredients:
- 6 frozen bananas
- ¼ cup nuts seeds

For the Topping:
- Syrup

Directions:
1. Fit an S-blade into your food processor. Process the bananas, a few pieces at a time. The bananas will start to break down into sections and cream. Keep adding the banana pieces until all the 6 bananas are over.
2. Whip until you get an ice cream-like texture but don't over-process, or the ice cream will be too soft. The pieces only need to break down. Scoop into a bowl, forming some balls. Splash with some nuts and top with syrup. Serve and enjoy!

Nutrition: Calories: 211 kcal, Protein: 7.8 g, Fiber: 5.0 g

191. Chocolate Peanut Butter Energy Bites

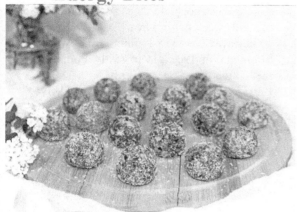

Preparation Time: 20 minutes, **Cooking Time:** 0 minutes, **Difficulty Level:** Easy, **Servings:** 4

Ingredients:
- ½ cup oats, old-fashioned
- ⅓ cup cocoa powder, unsweetened
- 1 cup dates, chopped
- ½ cup shredded coconut flakes, unsweetened
- ½ cup peanut butter

Directions:
1. Place oats in a food processor along with dates and pulse for 1 minute until the paste comes together.
2. Then add remaining ingredients, and blend until incorporated and a very thick mixture comes together.
3. Shape the mixture into balls, refrigerate for 1 hour until set, and serve.

Nutrition: Calories: 88.6 kcal, Fat: 5.0 g, Carbs: 10 g, Protein: 2.3 g, Fiber: 1.6 g

192. Cinnamon Berry Slush

Preparation Time: 10 minutes, **Cooking Time:** 0 minutes, **Difficulty Level:** Easy, **Servings:** 4

Ingredients:
- 1 cup frozen strawberries
- 1 cup apple, peeled and diced
- 2 tsp. fresh ginger
- 3 Tbsp. hemp seeds
- 1 cup water
- ½ lime juiced
- ¼ tsp. cinnamon powder
- ⅛ tsp. vanilla extract

Directions:
1. Add all the ingredients to a blender.
2. Blend well until smooth. Serve with fresh fruits

Nutrition: Calories: 144 kcal, Fat: 10 g, Fiber: 2.4 g

193. Cocoa Avocado Ice Cream

Preparation Time: 5 minutes, **Cooking Time:** 4 minutes, **Difficulty Level:** Moderate, **Serving:** 4

Ingredients:
- 1 can coconut milk, full fat
- 1 large ripe avocado, skin removed and pitted
- 3 Tbsp. raw cacao powder
- ¼ cup coconut nectar or agave
- ½ Tbsp. cinnamon
- 1 Tbsp. vanilla extract or powder

Directions:
1. Place all ingredients in a blender, high-speed, and process until a smooth consistency. Pour the mixture into a container, freezer friendly. Freeze for about 1 hour.
2. After 1 hour, continue to freeze for about 4 hours while whisking after every 30 minutes. This is to avoid freezer burn. Serve once the ice cream has thickened.

Nutrition: Calories: 144 kcal, Protein: 2.0 g, Fiber: 5.0 g

194. Coconut Raisins Cookies

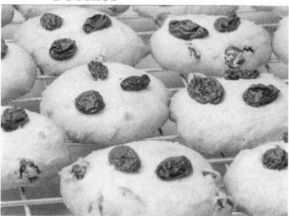

Preparation Time: 10 minutes, **Cooking Time:** 10 minutes, **Difficulty Level:** Moderate, **Servings:** 4

Ingredients:
- 1 ¼ cup almond flour
- 1 cup coconut flour
- 1 tsp. baking soda
- ½ tsp. Celtic sea salt
- 1 cup nut butter
- 1 cup coconut palm sugar
- 2 tsp. vanilla

- ¼ cup almond milk
- ¾ cup organic raisins
- ¾ cup coconut chips or flakes

Directions:
1. Set your oven to 357 °F. Mix flour with salt and baking soda. Blend butter with sugar until creamy, then stir in almond milk and vanilla.
2. Mix well, then stir in dry mixture. Mix until smooth. Fold in all the remaining ingredients. Make small cookies out of this dough.
3. Arrange the cookies on a baking sheet. Bake for 10 minutes until golden brown.

Nutrition: Calories: 237 kcal, Fat: 19.8 g, Protein: 17.8 g

195. Cranberry Refresher

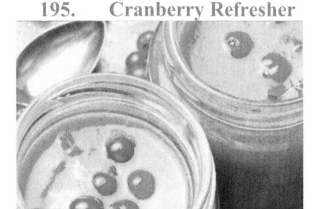

Preparation Time: 10 minutes, **Cooking Time:** 0 minutes, **Difficulty Level:** Easy, **Servings:** 4

Ingredients:
- 4 cup cranberries
- 3 cup almond milk
- 1 cup raspberries
- 8 tsp. fresh ginger, finely grated
- 8 tsp. fresh lemon juice

Directions:
1. Add all the ingredients to a blender.
2. Blend well until smooth. Serve with fresh berries on top.

Nutrition: Calories:146.6 kcal, Fat: 0.7 g, Fiber: 6.8 g

196. Crunchy Bars

Preparation Time: 5 minutes, **Cooking Time:** 5 minutes, **Difficulty Level:** Moderate, **Servings:** 4

Ingredients:
- 1 ½ cups sugar-free chocolate chips
- 1 cup almond butter
- Stevia, to taste
- ¼ cup coconut oil

- 3 cups pecans, chopped

Directions:
1. Layer an 8-inch baking pan with parchment paper. Mix chocolate chips with butter, coconut oil, and sweetener in a bowl. Melt it by heating in a microwave for 2 to 3 minutes until well mixed.
2. Stir in nuts and seeds. Mix gently. Pour batter into the baking pan. Spread evenly.
3. Refrigerate for 2 to 3 hours. Slice and serve.

Nutrition: Calories: 316 kcal, Sugar: 1.8 g, Fat: 30 g, Fiber: 3.8 g, Protein: 24 g

197. Green Tea Blueberry Shake

Preparation Time: 10 minutes, **Cooking Time:** 5 minutes, **Difficulty Level:** Easy, **Servings:** 4

Ingredients:
- 12 Tbsp. alkaline water
- 4 green tea bags
- 6 cups fresh blueberries
- 4 pears, peeled, cored, and diced
- 3 cups almond milk

Directions:
1. Boil 3 tablespoons of water in a small pot and transfer it to a cup. Dip the tea bag in the cup and let it sit for 4 to 5 minutes.
2. Discard the tea bag and transfer the green tea to a blender. Add all the remaining ingredients to the blender. Blend well until smooth. Serve with fresh blueberries.

Nutrition: Calories: 278 kcal, Fat: 2.97 g, Fiber: 10 g, Carbs: 65.4 g, Protein: 10.9 g

198. Homemade Coconut Ice Cream

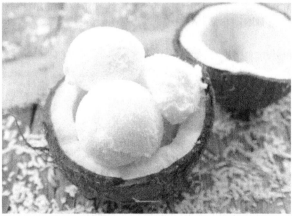

Preparation Time: 5 minutes, **Cooking Time:** 20 minutes, **Difficulty Level:** Hard, **Serving:** 4

Ingredients:
- 1 cup shredded coconut
- 1 Tbsp. vanilla
- 2 cans coconut milk, full fat
- 1 Tbsp. tapioca starch
- ½ cup coconut sugar

Directions:
1. Place ½ of the shredded coconut on a pan, then heat on a stove over medium-high heat for about 8-10 minutes until golden brown. Meanwhile, freeze a freezer bowl for a few hours before use.
2. Add vanilla, coconut milk, tapioca flour, and coconut sugar in a blender and process until smooth. Pour everything into the freezer bowl, then stir in the remaining shredded coconut.
3. Use manufacturer's instructions to set up your ice cream maker. This includes churning accordingly and adding your freezer bowl. Top with browned coconut and serve immediately.

Nutrition: Calories: 188 kcal, Protein: 1.0 g, Fiber: 1.0 g

199. Mango Coconut Cheesecake

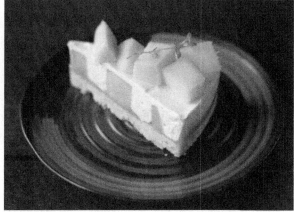

Preparation Time: 30 minutes, **Cooking Time:** 0 minutes, **Difficulty Level:** Moderate, **Servings:** 4

Ingredients:
For the Crust:
- 1 cup macadamia nuts
- 1 cup dates, pitted, soaked in hot water for 10 minutes

For the Filling:
- 1 Tbsp. and ½ cup maple syrup
- ⅓ cup and 2 Tbsp. coconut oil
- ¼ cup lemon juice
- 2 cups of cashews, soak in warm water for 10 minutes
- ½ cup and 2 Tbsp. coconut milk, unsweetened, chilled

For the Topping:
- 1 cup fresh mango slices

Directions:
1. Prepare the crust, and for this, place nuts in a food processor and process until mixture resembles crumbs.
2. Drain the dates, add them to the food processor and blend for 2 minutes until a thick mixture comes together.
3. Take a 4-inch cheesecake pan, place date mixture in it, spread and press evenly, and set aside.
4. Prepare the filling and for this, place all its ingredients in a food processor and blend for 3 minutes until smooth.
5. Pour the filling into the crust, spread evenly, and then freeze for 4 hours until set.
6. Top the cake with mango slices and then serve.

Nutrition: Calories: 200 kcal, Fat: 11.0 g, Carbs: 22.5 g, Protein: 2.0 g, Fiber: 1.0 g

200. Mini Berry Tarts

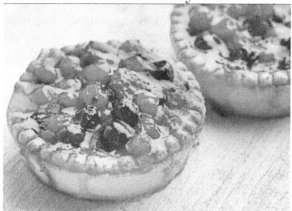

Preparation Time: 20 minutes, **Cooking Time:** 35 minutes, **Difficulty Level:** Hard, **Servings:** 4

Ingredients:
For the Pie Crust:
- ⅓ cup whole-wheat flour + more for dusting
- 4 Tbsp. flax seed powder
- 12 Tbsp. water
- ½ tsp. salt
- 3 Tbsp. pure malt syrup
- ¼ cup plant butter, cold and crumbled
- 1 ½ tsp. vanilla extract

For the Filling:
- 6 oz. cashew cream
- 6 Tbsp. pure date sugar
- ¾ tsp. vanilla extract
- 1 cup mixed frozen berries

Directions:

1. Preheat the oven to 350 °F. With cooking spray, grease a mini pie pan.
2. Mix the flaxseed powder with water in a medium bowl and allow soaking for 5 minutes.
3. Combine the flour and salt in a large bowl. Add the butter, and using an electric hand mixer, whisk until crumbly. Pour in the flax egg, malt syrup, vanilla, and mix until smooth dough forms.
4. Flatten the dough on a flat surface, cover with plastic wrap, and refrigerate for 1 hour.
5. After, lightly dust a working surface with some flour, remove the dough onto the surface, and using a rolling pin, flatten the dough into a 1-inch diameter circle,
6. Use a large cookie cutter, cut out rounds of the dough and fit into the pie pans. Use a knife to trim the edges of the pan. Lay a parchment paper on the dough cups, pour on some baking beans, and bake in the oven until golden brown, 15 to 20 minutes.
7. Remove the pans from the oven, pour out the baking beans, and allow cooling.
8. In a medium bowl, mix the cashew cream, date sugar, and vanilla extract.
9. Divide the mixture into the tart cups and top with berries. Serve immediately.

Nutrition: Calories: 358 kcal, Carbs: 33.5 g, Protein: 53.6 g, Protein: 10.6 g

201. Mixed Berry Mousse

Preparation Time: 10 minutes, **Cooking Time:** 25 minutes, **Difficulty Level:** Easy, **Servings:** 4

Ingredients:
- 1 tsp. lemon zest
- 3 oz. raspberries and blueberries
- ¼ tsp. vanilla essence
- 2 cups coconut cream

Directions:
1. Blend cream in an electric mixer until fluffy. Stir in vanilla and lemon zest. Mix well. Fold in nuts and berries.
2. Cover the bowl with plastic wrap. Refrigerate for 3 hours. Garnish as desired.

Nutrition: Calories: 265 kcal, Fat: 13.0 g, Fiber: 0.5 g

202. Peanut Butter Bars

Preparation Time: 10 minutes, **Cooking Time:** 10 minutes, **Difficulty Level:** Easy, **Servings:** 4

Ingredients:

- ¾ cup almond flour
- 2 oz. almond butter
- ¼ cup Swerve
- ½ cup peanut butter
- ½ tsp. vanilla

Directions:
1. Combine all the ingredients for bars. Transfer this mixture to a 6-inch small pan. Press it firmly.
2. Refrigerate for 30 minutes. Slice and serve.

Nutrition: Calories: 214 kcal, Fat: 19.0 g, Fiber: 2.1 g

203. Homemade Protein Bar

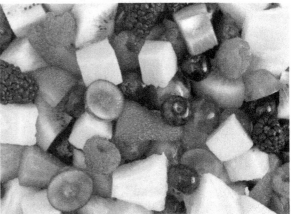

Preparation Time: 5 minutes, **Cooking Time:** 10 minutes, **Difficulty Level:** Easy, **Servings:** 4

Ingredients:
- 1 cup nut butter
- 4 Tbsp. coconut oil
- 2 scoops of vanilla protein
- Stevia, to taste
- ½ tsp. sea salt
- 1 tsp. cinnamon

Directions:
1. Mix coconut oil with butter, protein, stevia, and salt in a dish. Stir in the cinnamon and chocolate chips.
2. Press the mixture firmly and freeze until firm. Cut the crust into small bars. Serve and enjoy.

Nutrition: Calories: 179 kcal, Fat: 15.7 g, Sugar: 3.6 g

204.   Rainbow Fruit Salad

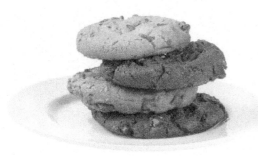

Preparation Time: 10 minutes, **Cooking Time:** 0 minutes, **Difficulty Level:** Moderate, **Servings:** 4

Ingredients:
For the Fruit Salad:
- 1 lb. strawberries, hulled, sliced
- 1 cup kiwis, halved or cubed
- 1 ¼ cups blueberries
- 1 ⅓ cups blackberries
- 1 cup pineapple chunks

For the Maple Lime Dressing:
- 2 tsp. lime zest
- ¼ cup maple syrup
- 1 Tbsp. lime juice

Directions:
1. Prepare the salad, and for this, take a bowl, place all its ingredients and toss until mixed.
2. Prepare the dressing, and for this, take a small bowl, place all its ingredients and whisk well.
3. Drizzle the dressing over salad, toss until coated, and serve.

Nutrition: Calories: 88.1 kcal, Fat: 0.4 g, Carbs: 22.6 g, Protein: 1.1 g, Fiber: 2.8 g

205.   Shortbread Cookies

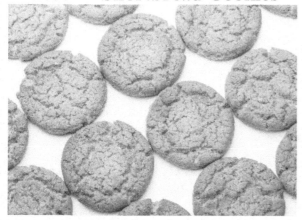

Preparation Time: 10 minutes, **Cooking Time:** 70 minutes, **Difficulty Level:** Moderate, **Servings:** 4

Ingredients:
- 2 ½ cups almond flour
- 6 Tbsp. nut butter
- ½ cup Erythritol
- 1 tsp. vanilla essence

Directions:
1. Preheat your oven to 350 °F. Layer a cookie sheet with parchment paper.
2. Beat butter with Erythritol until fluffy. Stir in vanilla essence and almond flour. Mix well until crumbly. Spoon out a Tbsp. of cookie dough onto the cookie sheet.
3. Add more dough to make as many cookies. Bake for 15 minutes until brown. Serve.

Nutrition: Calories: 288 kcal, Fat: 25.3 g, Fiber: 3.8 g

206.   Tropical Cookies
Preparation Time: 10 minutes, **Cooking Time:** 15 minutes, **Difficulty Level:** Moderate, **Servings:** 4

Ingredients:
- 1 cup almond flour
- ½ cup cacao nibs
- ½ cup coconut flakes, unsweetened
- ⅓ cup Erythritol
- ½ cup almond butter
- ¼ cup nut butter, melted
- ¼ cup almond milk
- Stevia, to taste
- ¼ tsp. sea salt

Directions:
1. Preheat your oven to 350 °F. Layer a cookie sheet with parchment paper. Add and combine the dry ingredients in a glass bowl.
2. Whisk in butter, almond milk, vanilla essence, Erythritol, and almond butter. Beat well, then stir in dry mixture. Mix well. Spoon out a tablespoon of cookie dough on the cookie sheet.
3. Add more dough to make as many as 16 cookies. Flatten each cookie using your fingers. Bake for 25 minutes until golden brown. Let them sit for 15 minutes. Serve.

Nutrition: Calories:192 kcal, Fat:17.44 g, Fiber: 2.1

Conclusion

When making the switch over to the plant-based eating plan, several benefits come to mind. While these benefits are not immediate, they do manifest themselves in a relatively short period. As such, patience is an important key when getting the most out of this new dietary approach.

The growing demand has been people trying out new recipes and mashing up ingredients in interesting ways. Have you heard of smoothies that contain cayenne pepper? It sounds pretty exciting, doesn't it? We are going to look at such wonderful and delicious recipes along with so many more dishes that use wholesome and natural ingredients.

Developing a practical plan will help you transition smoothly into a plant-based lifestyle. While doing this, you will also need your environment to support and focus on your diet plan. Your efforts should be directed towards learning more about this diet. For instance, you should subscribe to YouTube channels to watch and enjoy other vegan' videos as they delve into their experiences.

With all these recipes in this book, plus the tips given to you, I hope you find the plant-based diet easy to follow. However, without commitment, it will be impossible for you to achieve your set goals.

If you ever become bored with your diet, there is always something new to try! There are loads of whole foods for you to try in the world. You should never let the unknown intimidate you. Just give everything a try, and soon you will be building your perfect diet. By believing in yourself and making the right choices, you will be well on your way to a healthy and happy life.

Made in the USA
Monee, IL
29 March 2022

93728704R00063